KU-278-236

Contraception Today

A pocketbook for General Practitioners
Fourth edition

John Guillebaud
Medical Director
Margaret Pyke Centre
London, UK

MARTIN DUNITZ

© 2000 Martin Dunitz, an imprint of the Taylor & Francis Group

First published in the United Kingdom in 1992 as *Contraception: Hormonal and Barrier Methods* by
Martin Dunitz, an imprint of the Taylor and Francis Group, 11 New Fetter Lane, London EC4P 4EE

Tel.: +44 (0) 20 7583 9855
Fax.: +44 (0) 20 7842 2298
E-mail: info@dunitz.co.uk
Website: http://www.dunitz.co.uk

First edition 1992, reprinted 1993
Second edition 1995
Third edition 1997
Reprinted with revisions 1998, reprinted 1999
Fourth edition 2000, reprinted 2002

Although every effort has been made to ensure that drug doses and other information are presented accurately in this publication, the ultimate responsibility rests with the prescribing physician. Neither the publishers nor the authors can be held responsible for errors or for any consequences arising from the use of information contained herein. For detailed prescribing information or instructions on the use of any product or procedure discussed herein, please consult the prescribing information or instructional material issued by the manufacturer.

A CIP record for this book is available from the British Library.

ISBN 1–85317–868–3

Distributed in the USA by
Fulfilment Center
Taylor & Francis
10650 Tobben Drive
Independence, KY 41051, USA
Toll Free Tel.: +1 800 634 7064
E-mail: taylorandfrancis@thomsonlearning.com

Distributed in Canada by
Taylor & Francis
74 Rolark Drive
Scarborough, Ontario M1R 4G2, Canada
Toll Free Tel.: +1 877 226 2237
E-mail: tal_fran@istar.ca

Distributed in the rest of the world by
Thomson Publishing Services
Cheriton House
North Way
Andover, Hampshire SP10 5BE, UK
Tel.: +44 (0)1264 332424
E-mail: salesorder.tandf@thomsonpublishingservices.co.uk

Composition by Wearset Ltd, Boldon, Tyne and Wear

Printed and bound in Italy by Printer Trento

Contents

Preface

> *Family planning could bring more benefits to more people at less cost than any other single 'technology' now available to the human race.*
>
> UNICEF

Recalling that every new birth in the UK is likely in its life-time to do as much damage to the environment as 30–200 births in Burundi or Bangladesh will ever have the chance to do, this quote applies worldwide. So I welcome the opportunity to produce this pocketbook for general practitioners on the subject of contraception.

I write as one who is proud to have worked in general practice, as a locum in places as diverse as Barnsley, Cambridge, Luton and South London, and is hence able to appreciate some of the constraints of that role.

March 2000

Introduction

General practitioners (GPs) are often well placed to offer good contraceptive advice because they already know the patient's health and circumstances. Some practices are excellent; others provide little beyond oral contraception and devote insufficient time and skill to counselling. Ideally there should be at least one dedicated family planning session each week to deal with first visits and methods such as intrauterine devices (IUDs) or systems (IUSs) and implants. Women raising more complex contraceptive problems may be asked to reattend, after the surgery. Much can, indeed should, be delegated to a practice nurse fully trained in family planning, usually with a gain rather than a loss in standards. The following may be appropriately delegated to her:

- Taking sexual and medical history, discussion of choices
- Cap fitting, checking, teaching
- Pill teaching
- Pill reissuing, and emergency pill issuing against an agreed protocol. (At present UK law does not permit appropriately trained nurses to *prescribe* contraceptive hormones, but hopefully this will change)
- Pill monitoring in the absence of risk factors
- IUD and IUS checking
- Cervical smear taking

The practice nurse should also be taught to detect, and then always seek advice for, the simple but important sign of cervical excitation tenderness.

Formal training is also desirable for doctors* and should include both theoretical and 'apprenticeship' training, as well as discussion of the often complex psychosexual and emotional factors involved in the use of contraception. All clinicians should be sensitive to hidden signals in this area.

Doctors should back their counselling with good literature. Although some manufacturers have improved their package labelling, the latest UK Family Planning Association leaflets are better — 'user-friendly', yet accurate and comprehensive. *Your Guide to Contraception* tabulates all the important methods, both reversible and permanent, and is ideal for reading in the waiting room before counselling. The leaflets on individual methods, especially *Choosing and Using the Combined Pill*, should be given with advice to 'read, and keep long term for further reference'. Its month and date of publication should be recorded in the patient's notes. Follow-up patients may need a replacement. Together with accurate contemporary records, these leaflets provide strong medicolegal back-up for practitioners who may be asked to justify their actions in the event of litigation. They are an essential supplement to — but by no means a replacement for — time spent with the doctor and/or nurse.

Choice of method

Most women who seek contraception are healthy and young, and present fewer problems than the over-35s, teenagers and those with intercurrent disease. There is an increasing tendency for sterilization procedures to be demanded at too early an age. This is partly because the pill is too often seen as synonymous with contraception,

---

* In the UK, the Faculty of Family Planning and Reproductive Health Care offers, through agencies such as the Margaret Pyke Centre (MPC), educational courses leading to their Diploma (DFFP) and Membership (MFFP), as well as a range of Letters of Competence. The Institute of Psychosexual Medicine offers relevant seminar training.

and we as providers have not been informing women about the many new or improved reversible alternatives to the pill and condom, about which there is still much ignorance and mythology. I refer particularly to the levonorgestrel intra-uterine system (LNG IUS), the GyneT380, the GyneFix, injectables and the latest implants.

The very young

Although early cycles after the menarche are assumed to be anovulatory, very early conceptions are increasingly reported, and surveys show that around half the total female population aged 16 years or under have had inter-course. Easier access to emergency contraception is an obvious priority. As they may often 'get away with it' in one or more cycles, however, all too often the young do not seek advice until they have already conceived. Education must therefore promote (as in The Netherlands) the societal norm that sex may be a feature of a good relationship only when and if adequate contraception exists. In this age group we still await as first-line more 'forgettable' methods in which (in contrast to pills) non-pregnancy is the 'default state'. Injectables and implants are preferable to copper IUDs, because they provide some protection against pelvic infection, although IUDs are only relatively contraindicated (the GyneFix or LNG IUS may be appropriate).

In spite of not having the ideal 'default state', for many young women the most suitable initial method currently remains a modern, low-oestrogen, combined oral contra-ceptive (COC), backed by good counselling. Once periods have been established there appear to be no special medical problems of the pill for teenagers, as compared with women in their early 20s.

With patients under 16 the GP should, merely as part of good medical practice — so long as it is done opportunely, non-judgementally and in a non-patronizing way — present the emotional, physical and legal advantages of delaying intercourse (and then of mutual loyalty). But the 'best' must not become the enemy of the 'good', a category that surely includes contraception (with age-appropriate sexual health education) when the foregoing is rejected. Involvement of at least one parent is vastly preferable, yet it can be good practice to prescribe the pill without it (see Box). *At all times the young woman must be assured of confidentiality.*

There is a useful mnemonic for the UK Memorandum of Guidance (DHSS HC(FP)86), issued after the Gillick case:

Mnemonic: UnProtected SSexual InterCourse. The doctor:

U Must ensure the young person UNDERSTANDS the potential risks and benefits of the treatment/advice given

P Is legally obliged to discuss the value of PARENTAL support, yet the client must know that confidentiality is respected whether or not this is given

S Should assess whether the client is likely to have SEXUAL INTERCOURSE without contraception

S Should assess whether the young person's physical/mental health may SUFFER if not given contraceptive advice or supplies

I Must consider if it is in the client's best INTERESTS to give contraception without parental consent

C Must respect the duty of CONFIDENTIALITY that should be given to a person under 16, and which is as great as that owed to any other person

HIV and other sexually transmitted infections

No opportunity should be missed to advise the sexually active of all ages on minimizing their risk of sexually transmitted infections (STIs), including the human immunodeficiency virus (HIV). Besides 'selling' monogamy — on medical grounds — *it is essential to promote the condom as an addition to the selected contraceptive whenever infection risk exists: the so-called Double Dutch approach.*

Relative effectiveness of available methods

Good results depend on a couple-based, individualized approach — contraception is very much about choosing 'horses for courses'. Iatrogenic pregnancies can frequently be caused by omissions and errors on the part of service providers — and these are by definition avoidable. Table 1 outlines the comparative efficacy of most current methods.

Unwanted effects of contraceptives: contraindications

These are obviously important issues, but risks must be impartially evaluated (a failing of the mass media) and then rationally applied as contraindications (a failing often of doctors, who tend to introduce unnecessary medical barriers to contraceptive use).

An important general principle is *summation*, discussed on p. 36. Also important is the WHO system for classifying contraindications, which is applied in this book (to the best of my judgement). It is evidence-based, where evidence exists, but also tries to give the best interim guidance when we have to make a decision (in consultation with the woman/couple), in the frustrating absence of good evidence. This scheme (which I had a hand in devising at a WHO meeting in Atlanta, 1994) is more fully described in a 1996 WHO document on medical eligibility criteria (WHO/FRH/FPP96.9).

Table 1
First-year user-failure rates/100 women for different methods of contraception.

Method of contraception	Range in the world literature*	Oxford/FPA study (Lancet report in 1982; all women married and aged above 25)	
		Age 25–34 (≤2 years' use)	Age 35+ (≤2 years' use)
Sterilization			
Male (after azoospermia)	0–0.05	0.08	0.08
Female	0–0.5	0.45	0.08
Subcutaneous implant			
Implanon	0–0.07		
Injectable (DMPA)	0–1	–	–
Combined pills			
50 µg oestrogen	0.1–3	0.25	0.17
<50 µg oestrogen	0.2–3	0.38	0.23
Progestogen-only pill	0.3–4	2.5	0.5
IUD			
Nova-T	1–2		
Nova-T380	0.6		
Multiload Cu 375	0.2–1		
Gyne T380	0.2–1		
Levonorgestrel IUS	0.1–0.2		
Diaphragm	4–20	5.5	2.8
(Male) condom	2–15	6.0	2.9
Female condom	5–15		
Coitus interruptus	6–17	–	–
Spermicides alone	4–25	–	–
Fertility awareness	2–25	–	–
'Persona'	6–?	–	–
No method, young women	80–90	–	–
No method at age 40	40–50	–	–
No method at age 45	10–20	–	–
No method at age 50 (if still having menses)	0–5	–	–

*Excludes atypical studies and all extended use studies. For sterilization, rates in first column are estimated **lifetime failure rates**

Note: 1 First figure of range in first column gives a rough measure of 'perfect use' (but is not the same)

    2 Influence of age, all the rates in the fourth column being lower than those in the third column. Lower rates still may be expected above age 45

    3 Much better results also obtainable in other states of relative infertility, such as lactation

    4 Oxford/FPA users were established users as recruitment – greatly improving results especially for barrier methods

There are now four categories of contraindication:

WHO Classification of contraindications*
1. A condition for which there is no restriction for the use of the contraceptive method
   'A' is for **ALWAYS USABLE**
2. A condition where the advantages of the method generally outweigh the theoretical or proven risks
   'B' is for **BROADLY USABLE**
3. A condition where the theoretical or proven risks usually outweigh the advantages. But — respecting the patient/client's autonomy — if she accepts the risks and rejects or should not use relevant alternatives, the method can be used with caution/additional care — as a 'method of last choice'
   'C' is for **CAUTION/COUNSELLING**, if used at all
4. A condition which represents an unacceptable health risk
   'D' is for **DO NOT USE**, at all

---

* My A–B–C–D additions are just aide-mémoires. WHO 1–2–3–4 numbering is used in the book, to avoid confusion.

The most useful new feature of the classification is the separation into two categories of RELATIVE contraindication (categories 2 and 3).

Clinical judgement is required in consultation with the contraceptive user when deciding whether to use the method, especially in all category 3 conditions, or if more than one category 3 or 2 condition applies (usually then signifies 4, 'Do not use').

Combined oral contraceptives

Mechanism of action

Aside from secondary contraceptive effects on the cervical mucus and to impede implantation, COCs primarily prevent ovulation. They therefore 'remove' the normal menstrual cyle and replace it with a cycle which is user-produced and based only on the end-organ, the endometrium. So the withdrawal bleeding has minimal medical significance, can be deliberately postponed or made infrequent as in tri-cycling (see below), and if it fails to occur, once pregnancy is excluded, poses 'no problem'. The pill-free time is the contraception-deficient time, which has great relevance to maintenance of the COC's efficacy (see below).

Benefits versus risks

COCs can provide virtually 100% protection from unwanted pregnancy. They can be taken at a time unconnected with intercourse and provide enormous reassurance by the regular, short, light and usually painless withdrawal bleed-ing at the end of each pack. Most of the discussion here concerns possible risks*, but the positive aspects should not be forgotten.

Contraceptive benefits of COCs
- Effectiveness
- Convenience, not intercourse-related
- Reversibility

Non-contraceptive benefits of COCs
- Reduction of most menstrual cycle disorders: less heavy bleeding, therefore less anaemia, and less dysmenorrhoea; regular bleeding, and timing can be controlled (no pill-taker need have 'periods' at weekends); fewer symptoms of premenstrual tension overall; no ovulation pain
- Fewer functional ovarian cysts because abnormal ovulation prevented
- Fewer extrauterine pregnancies because normal ovulation inhibited
- Reduction in pelvic inflammatory disease (PID)
- Reduction in benign breast disease
- Fewer symptomatic fibroids
- Probable reduction in thyroid disease (both overactive and underactive syndromes)
- Probable reduction in risk of rheumatoid arthritis
- Fewer sebaceous disorders (with oestrogen-dominant COCs)
- Possibly fewer duodenal ulcers (not well established and perhaps due to avoidance of COCs by anxious women)
- Reduction in *Trichomonas vaginalis* infections
- Possible lower incidence of toxic shock syndrome
- Beneficial effect on cancers of ovary and endometrium (see text)
- No toxicity in overdose
- Obvious beneficial social effects

* Data derived mainly from the prospective Royal College of General Practitioners (RCGP), Oxford/Family Planning Association (FPA) and US Nurses Studies, supplemented by numerous case–control studies conducted by WHO and other bodies.

Even as we turn to unwanted effects, it is reassuring that, according to the RCGP report in 1999, COCs have their main (small) effect on every known cause of mortality during current use and for some (variable) time thereafter. The excess thrombotic risk has probably vanished by 4 weeks, and, by 10 years after use ceases, mortality in past users is indistinguishable from that in never users.

Tumours

Breast cancer

This has a high incidence and therefore it must inevitably be expected to develop in women whether they take COCs or not. As the recognized risk factors for breast cancer include early menarche and late age of first birth, use of COCs by young women is bound to receive scientific scrutiny. However, if there is a real causative link with pill use, use by older women will obviously lead to more attributable cases as the incidence rises steeply above age 35 years (Figure 1). The literature to date is copious, complex, confusing and contradictory. Research is complicated by the problems related to possible latency, changes in formulation, time of exposure and high-risk groups.

The 1996 publication by the Collaborative Group on Hormonal Factors in Breast Cancer (CGHFBC) proposed a new model which is the one now most widely accepted. The group reanalysed original data from over 53 000 women with breast cancer and over 100 000 controls from 54 studies in 25 countries. This is 90% of the worldwide epidemiological data.

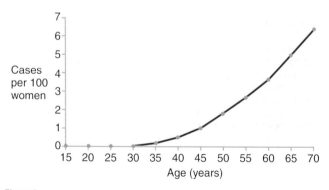

Figure 1
Background risk: cumulative number of breast cancers per 100 women, by age.
(Reproduced from statement by Faculty of Family Planning, June 1996.)

Previously the most widely accepted view was that the increased risk associated with the pill was for breast cancer occurring at a young age, and that it diminished or disappeared at older ages — that is, the risk is transient. The CGHFBC's model shows disappearance of the risk in ex-users, but now 'recency of use' of the COC is the most important factor, with the odds ratio unaffected by age of initiation or discontinuation, use before or after first full-term pregnancy, or duration of use. The main findings are summarized in Table 2.

Table 2
The increased risk of developing breast cancer while taking the pill and in the 10 years after stopping (CGHFBC 1996).

User status	Increased risk
Current user	24%
1–4 years after stopping	16%
5–9 years after stopping	7%
10 plus years an ex-user	No significant excess

COC users can be reassured that:

- While the small increase in breast cancer risk for women on the pill noted in previous studies is confirmed, the odds ratio of 1.24 signifies an increase of 24% only while women are taking the COC and for a few years thereafter, diminishing to zero after 10 years
- Beyond 10 years after stopping there is no detectable increase in breast cancer risk for former pill users. (Professor Klim McPherson of London is among those who highlight a continuing doubt that this will be true for women exposed for a long duration before their first full-term pregnancy. Fortunately this potential latency concern causes less anxiety to other authorities, as more data are acquired)
- The cancers diagnosed in women who use or have ever used COCs are clinically less advanced than in those who have never used the pill, and are less likely to have spread beyond the breast
- This re-analysis shows that these risks are not associated with duration of use or the dose or type of hormone in the COC, and that there is no synergism with other risk factors for breast cancer (e.g. family history, see text)
- The apparent risk for users of progestogen-only contraceptives (POP and injectable) was similar to the COC, but failed to reach statistical significance

The collaborative group conceded that its findings in ever-takers of the pill, of less advanced cases being identified but more of them at each given age, suggested surveillance bias — and the latter might even explain all or part of the findings in current users as well. However, the consensus interpretation which I personally accept for the present is that the pill is a weak co-factor for breast cancer, but that for some reason the resulting tumours are less aggressive.

Clinical implications

The Faculty of Family Planning in the UK states that pill-users should be informed of/counselled about the above data, but reiterates the advice of the UK Committee on the Safety of Medicines that there need be no fundamental change in prescribing practice.

The breast cancer issue should now normally be addressed, in a sensitive way, as part of routine pill counselling for all women. This discussion should be initiated opportunely — not necessarily at the first visit if not raised by the woman — along with encouragement to report promptly any unusual changes in the breasts at any time in the future ('breast awareness'). The balancing protective effects against malignancy of the ovary and endometrium (see below) should also be mentioned. *The known contraceptive and non-contraceptive benefits of COCs may seem so great to many (but not to all) as to compensate for almost any likely lifetime excess risk of breast cancer*.

Figure 2 helps to summarize the situation. Imagine a concert hall (Hall 1) filled with 1000 pill-users, all *now aged 45*, but all having used the COC for varying durations of time, then *having stopped by age 35* (a common situation). The (cumulative) number of cases of breast cancer would be 11. However, in a similar auditorium (Hall 2) filled with never-takers of the pill also all aged 45 there would be 10 cases — i.e. there is only one pill-attributable case, allowing

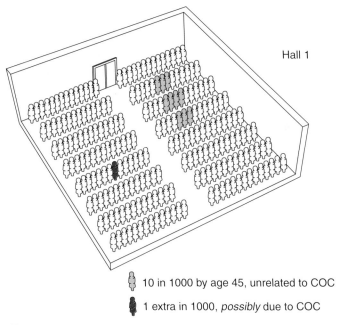

Hall 1

🧍 10 in 1000 by age 45, unrelated to COC

🧍 1 extra in 1000, *possibly* due to COC

Figure 2
Cumulative incidence of breast cancer during and after use of COC until age 35.

for pill use of any duration to age 35 plus 10 years' ex-use.
Moreover:

- If the pill is acting as a co-factor for breast cancer it is possible that the one excess case is a woman who would have developed the disease without the pill anyway, but at a later age
- The remaining 989 ex-pill-users will from this time on have only the same risk of breast cancer as other women now aged 45 — i.e. there is no ongoing added risk, because it is over 10 years since their last pill. This is a very important finding given that the overall risk of breast cancer rises so much with age (see also p. 9)
- The cancers diagnosed among the pill-users in Hall 1, already and in future, will tend to be less advanced than those in Hall 2

What about pill use by the *older woman*? Or, in *high-risk groups for breast cancer*, specifically (a) women with a family history of a young (under 40) first-degree relative with breast cancer and (b) women with benign breast disease (BBD) *without* pre-malignant epithelial atypia on histology? (If present, the latter is WHO 4: avoid COC.)

Older women are now permitted to use the COC to age 50 if they so choose, provided they are healthy, migraine-free non-smokers. The cumulative risk of breast cancer in young women is very small, being 1 in 500 in women up to age 35. However, the cumulative risk increases with age thereafter, to 1 in 100 at age 45 and 1 in 12 by age 75. *If the background risk for the individual is larger, whether because of increased age, uncomplicated BBD or a family history*, the percentage increment (24%) during current use does not increase. However, *applied to a bigger background risk* (see Figure 1) *it will obviously mean more attributable cases* (than in younger women without any risk factors for breast cancer). Therefore, these are **relative contraindications** (usually WHO 2), requiring careful explanation. If the woman chooses the COC — as she is entitled to do, given its contraceptive advantages and protection against cancer of the ovary and endometrium (see below) — it should be a low-dose formulation, with specific counselling, extra surveillance and periodic reassessment.

If carcinoma of the breast develops, the prognosis is good in pill-users; however, COCs should be stopped. Progestogen-only methods are an option after consultation with the woman's oncologist.

Cervical cancer
In 1983, and again in 1996, the Oxford/FPA study showed a significant increase in cervical neoplasia in long-term COC-users compared with IUD users. The UK RCGP study found that for current and recent users compared prospectively with the non-using controls, the odds ratio for mortality was

2.5, significantly raised. In that study of 46 000 women the non-users were materially different people, however, with a greater use of barrier methods, and their sexual lifestyles may well have differed. The association is not in doubt, but causality is less clear.

Studies of cervical cancer are always complicated by a lack of accurate information on sexual activity of women and especially their partners. The principal carcinogen is clearly transmitted sexually and is probably a virus or combination of viruses. COCs may act as weak co-factors (certainly weaker than cigarette smoking), and there are suggestive data that they may speed transition through the later pre-invasive stages.

Clinical implications

1. Prescribers must of course ensure that pill-users are screened following agreed guidelines. The higher mortality of COC-users in the RCGP study ought to be avoidable in future, now that computerized recall and agreed targets in the UK are ensuring the inclusion in screening of high-risk groups who were missed before, and subsequent early treatment of pre-invasive lesions.
2. It is acceptable practice (WHO 1–2) to continue COC use during the careful monitoring of any abnormality, or after definitive treatment of cervical intraepithelial neoplasia (CIN).

Liver tumours

COC use increases the relative risk of **benign adenoma** or **hamartoma**, and they can cause pain or a haemoperitoneum. However, the background incidence is so small (1–3 per 1 million women per year) that the COC-attributable risk is minimal. Most reported cases have been in long-term users of relatively high-dose pills.

Three case–control studies support the view that **primary hepatocellular carcinoma** (without any apparent synergism with cirrhosis or hepatitis B infection) is less rare in COC-users than it is in controls. If the link is causative the maximum attributable incidence would be about 4 per million users per year (Vessey 1989).

Choriocarcinoma

UK studies (but not others in the USA) have shown that chemotherapy for choriocarcinoma is more often required among women given COCs in the presence of active trophoblastic disease.

Clinical implications

1. When any form of trophoblastic disease has been diagnosed, therefore, in the UK the Regional Centres which monitor all cases still strongly recommend that sex steroids should be avoided while human chorionic gonadotrophin (hCG) levels are raised. This advice includes the progestogen-only methods, but emergency contraception is permitted: WHO 3.
2. What contraception until hCG is undetectable? Fortunately, while hCG levels are above 5000 iu/l ovulation is very improbable so barrier methods should be effective. Copper IUDs are usable, after preliminary imaging to exclude invasive damage to the uterine wall from cancer.

Carcinomas of the ovary and of the endometrium

The good news is that both are definitely less frequent in COC-users. Numerous studies have shown that the incidence of both is roughly halved among all users, and reduced to one-third in long-term users; a protective effect can be detected in ex-users for up to 10–15 years. Suppression of ovulation and of normal menstruation in COC-users probably explains these findings.

Other cancers

Other links with cancer (e.g. possible protection against colorectal cancer) have been mooted but not confirmed.

Benefits and risks — a summary for cancer

In counselling, a balance needs to be found (Figure 3). It has been concluded on the basis of computer modelling that populations using COCs may develop different benign or malignant neoplasms from control populations, but there is no proof that the overall risk of neoplasia is increased (it could even be reduced, although there is no proof of that either).

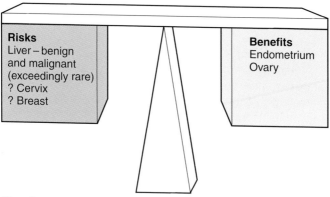

Figure 3
Cancer and COCs: a balance.

Circulatory disease and choice of COC

The objective of prescribing is efficacy with maximum safety, and with the pill this primarily means safety in relation to arterial and venous circulatory disease. This safety depends on choosing appropriate users as much as appropriate pills. The following is a useful framework for this process:

1. What are the benefits versus the risks? (Discussed above, and pp. 25–27)
2. Who should never take the pill? (The **absolute contraindications**, pp. 33–34)
3. Who usually should not take the pill? Maybe, but then with special advice, alertness to synergism and monitoring (the relative contraindications, pp. 28, 29, 35)

Among these, risk factors for circulatory disease are of greatest relevance, and the research available since 1995 means we should now consider *separately* for each woman the risk factors for venous and arterial thrombosis. Questions (2) and (3) identify the least and the less 'safe' women for each of these types of circulatory problem, and the answers are pivotal in the next choice for each category, namely:

4. Which are the safer pills?

All modern low-dose COCs contain ethinyloestradiol (EE) combined with a variety of progestogens, as in Figure 4 and Table 3. (Note that there are only five main 'ladders' of progestogens, since *in vivo* norethisterone acetate is converted with great efficiency to norethisterone.) These progestogens are classified into two groups, often but unhelpfully referred to as 'second generation' (levonorgestrel [LNG] and norethisterone [NET] with its prodrugs) or 'third generation' (desogestrel [DSG] and gestodene [GSD]). Norgestimate does not fit comfortably into either group (see p. 33).

The type of risk factor present (venous or arterial) and her experience during previous use by that woman determine the type of progestogen chosen. The intention is to minimize adverse effects of both pill components, by giving the lowest acceptable dose of the oestrogen and allowing for differences in known biological effects of the progestogens. In simple terms, smaller pills give smaller side effects.

5. Which second choice of pill?

This particularly means accounting for individual variation in pharmacology, and endometrial bleeding as a possible biological 'assay' of the contraceptive steroids (see pp. 38–39).

Table 3 Formulations of currently marketed combined oral contraceptives (COCs).

Pill type	Preparation	Oestrogen (µg)	Progestogen (µg)
Monophasic			
Ethinyloestradiol/ norethisterone type	Loestrin 20	20	1000 Norethisterone acetate*
	Loestrin 30	30	1500 Norethisterone acetate*
	Brevinor	35	500 Norethisterone
	Ovysmen	35	500 Norethisterone
	Norimin	35	1000 Norethisterone
Ethinyloestradiol/ levonorgestrel	Microgynon 30 (also ED)	30	150
	Ovranette	30	150
	Eugynon 30	30	250
	Ovran 30	30	250
	Ovran	50	250
Ethinyloestradiol/ desogestrel	Mercilon	20	150
	Marvelon	30	150
Ethinyloestradiol/ gestodene	Femodene (also ED)	30	75
	Minulet	30	75
Ethinyloestradiol/ norgestimate	Cilest	35	250
Mestranol/ norethisterone	Norinyl-1	50	1000
Bi/triphasic			
Ethinyloestradiol/ norethisterone	BiNovum	35	500 ⎱ 833† (7 tabs)
		35	1000 ⎰ (14 tabs)
	Synphase	35	500 ⎱ (7 tabs)
		35	1000 ⎬ 714 (9 tabs)
		35	500 ⎰ (5 tabs)
	TriNovum	35	500 ⎱ (7 tabs)
		35	750 ⎬ 750 (7 tabs)
		35	1000 ⎰ (7 tabs)
Ethinyloestradiol/ levonorgestrel	Logynon (also ED)	30 ⎱	50 (6 tabs)
		40 ⎬ 32†	75 ⎬ 92 (5 tabs)
		30 ⎰	125 (10 tabs)
	Trinordiol	30 ⎱	50 (6 tabs)
		40 ⎬ 32	75 ⎬ 92 (5 tabs)
		30 ⎰	125 (10 tabs)
Ethinyloestradiol/ gestodene	Tri-Minulet	30 ⎱	50 (6 tabs)
		40 ⎬ 32	70 ⎬ 79 (5 tabs)
		30 ⎰	100 (10 tabs)
	Triadene	30 ⎱	50 (6 tabs)
		40 ⎬ 32	70 ⎬ 79 (5 tabs)
		30 ⎰	100 (10 tabs)
New formulations **Monophasic brand**			
Ethinyloestradiol/ levonorgestrel	Microgynon 20 ‡	20	100
Ethinyloestradiol/ gestodene	Femodette	20	75
Biphasic			
Ethinyloestradiol/ desogestrel	Gracial ‡	40 ⎱ 33	25 ⎱ 93 (7 tabs)
		30 ⎰	125 ⎰ (15 tabs)

*Converted to norethisterone as the active metabolite.
†Equivalent daily doses for comparison with monophasic brands.
‡Not available at the time of writing, likely to become available shortly.
Other names are on pp. 116–118.

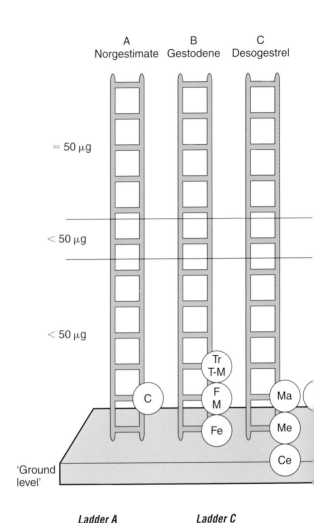

Figure 4
COC formulations available in the UK. Note: ED or every day means placebos are given on pill-free days.

Ladder A
C = Cilest
Ladder B
Tr = Triadene
T-M = Tri-Minulet
F = Femodene (also ED)
M = Minulet
Fe = Femodette

Ladder C
G = Gracial
Ma = Marvelon
Me = Mercilon
Ce = Cerazette
Ladder D
Ov = Ovran
O30 = Ovran 30
E30 = Eugynon 30
Oe = Ovranette

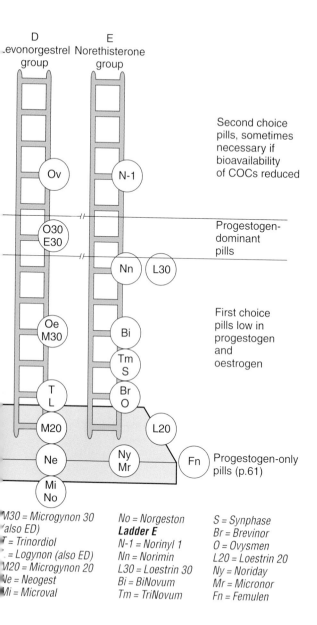

D
Levonorgestrel group

E
Norethisterone group

Second choice pills, sometimes necessary if bioavailability of COCs reduced

Ov

N-1

Progestogen-dominant pills

O30
E30

Nn   L30

First choice pills low in progestogen and oestrogen

Oe
M30

Bi

Tm
S

T
L

Br
O

M20

L20

Ne

Ny
Mr

Fn   Progestogen-only pills (p.61)

Mi
No

M30 = Microgynon 30 (also ED)
T = Trinordiol
L = Logynon (also ED)
M20 = Microgynon 20
Ne = Neogest
Mi = Microval

No = Norgeston
Ladder E
N-1 = Norinyl 1
Nn = Norimin
L30 = Loestrin 30
Bi = BiNovum
Tm = TriNovum

S = Synphase
Br = Brevinor
O = Ovysmen
L20 = Loestrin 20
Ny = Noriday
Mr = Micronor
Fn = Femulen

21

This includes:

- The implications of the pill-free week
- Blood pressure
- Headaches, especially migraines
- Management of important new risk factors or diseases
- Management of 'minor' side effects

Venous thromboembolism and arterial wall disease

The dust has at last settled on the media hype and 'pill scare' which followed a letter from the UK Committee on the Safety of Medicines (CSM) on 18 October 1995, based on three congruent but at the time unpublished studies. At the time many of us wished that the story had been officially presented as a *reduction* of risk of venous thrombo-embolism (VTE) if women used LNG or NET pills. I see this as not just a matter of presentation (explaining to the public and the media that 'the bottle is half full, rather than half empty'). It is also scientifically more valid. This is because the *different* progestogen is really levonorgestrel, which behaves anti-oestrogenically in many of its biological effects. We have known for years that LNG tends to oppose the oestrogen-mediated rise in sex hormone binding globulin (SHBG) and high density lipoprotein (HDL) cholesterol (and even lowers the latter if enough is given). It also opposes the tendency for oestrogen to improve acne. It is thus unlike DSG and GSD, which basically both allow oestrogen to 'do its own thing'.

A major study at the Margaret Pyke Centre compared the four main progestogens (DSG, GSD, LNG and NET) combined with the same 30 µg dose of EE. We confirmed the above biochemical differences between the two types of progestogen and the fact that NET is similar to, but less potent than, LNG in opposing at least some of the effects of oestrogen (Figure 5).

Researchers from The Netherlands and the UK are at the time of writing beginning to identify differences in the haemostatic system among users of DSG- or GSD- compared with LNG-containing pills, which could explain a difference in thrombotic risk, favouring the latter pills.

Accordingly, it is no longer 'biologically implausible' that the combination of LNG with EE reduces the prothrombotic (oestrogenic) effects of EE below what they would be with 30 μg EE alone. Why should DSG and GSD not simply fail to have that opposing action, just as they do when we actually want a greater oestrogenic effect (e.g. when choosing a pill for someone with acne)?

However, the apparent halving of the risk shown in four studies is likely to be an exaggeration of any beneficial effect of LNG and NET on VTE risk. This is because of the well-established influence of prescriber bias and the so-called healthy user effect in all the studies (leading to LNG/NET pill use being more probable in women at lower intrinsic risk, and vice versa). There have also been negative studies since 1995, by Farmer, Lidegaard and others. In my opinion a real difference in VTE risk probably exists, but the ratio is likely to be lower than 2:1 — which makes it a small enough difference (particularly in absolute terms — see Table 4 and Figure 6) for many women to disregard it.

Does the apparent 'biological oestrogenicity' of DSG/GSD pills make them relatively better than LNG/NET pills for arterial wall diseases, especially acute myocardial infarction (AMI)? The Transnational Study (1997) found a statistically lower risk of AMI with DSG/GSD pills than with LNG pills (odds ratio 0.3, 95% CI 0.1–0.9), as was predicted from previous data on lipids and by analogy with HRT. However, it

A) SHBG increment

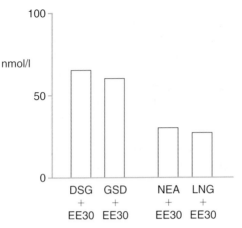

B) HDL cholesterol changes

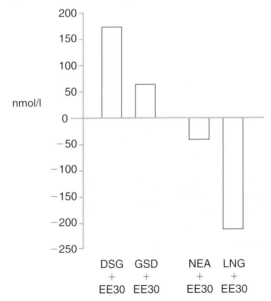

Figure 5
A) Prospective RCT of 4 pills: SHBG increment (MPC). B) Prospective RCT of 4 pills: HDL cholesterol changes (MPC)

appears that that study's finding may in fact be explained by inadequate screening for hypertension in older users of LNG/NET pills. Moreover, in the WHO study (1998) no difference in risk was found after controlling for measurement of blood pressure (which is, of course, a surrogate for good care). All other epidemiology to date indicates that if there is an arterial wall advantage through taking DSG/GSD pills it can only exist among pill-takers with arterial risk factors. See further pp. 31–32.

The advice in a Press Release (7 April 1999) from the Department of Health (DoH) issued after the 1998 review by

Table 4
Comparative risks – estimates 1996.

Annual risks per 100 000 women

Activity	Cases	Deaths
Having a baby, UK (all causes of death)		6
Having a baby (venous thromboembolism [VTE])	60	1
Using DSG/GSD pill (VTE)	25	<1 (0.4)
Using LNG/NET pill (VTE)	15	<1 (0.25)
Non-user, non-pregnant (VTE)	5–11	<1 (0.1)
		Mortality is 1–2%
Risk from **all causes** through COC (healthy non-smoking woman)		1
Home accidents		3
Playing soccer		4
Road accidents		8
Parachuting (10 jumps/year)		20
Scuba diving		22
Hang-gliding		150
Cigarette smoking (in next year if aged 35)		167
Death from pregnancy/ childbirth in rural Africa		1000 plus

Sources: Dinman B D (1980) *JAMA* **244**: 1226–8; Mills A et al (1996) *BMJ* **312**: 121; Anon (1991) *BMJ* **302**: 743. Strom B *Pharmacoepidemiology* 2nd edn (Chichester: Wiley, 1994): 57–65.

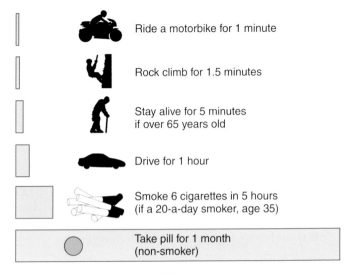

Ride a motorbike for 1 minute

Rock climb for 1.5 minutes

Stay alive for 5 minutes
if over 65 years old

Drive for 1 hour

Smoke 6 cigarettes in 5 hours
(if a 20-a-day smoker, age 35)

Take pill for 1 month
(non-smoker)

Time

Figure 6
Time required to have a 1:1 000 000 risk of dying. (Adapted from Minerva, British Medical Journal, 1988.)

the Medicines Commission of the VTE issue raised by the CSM in October 1995 'found no new safety concerns' about third generation DSG or gestodene GSD products.

'An increased risk of venous thromboembolic disease (VTE) associated with the use of oral contraceptives is well established but is smaller than that associated with pregnancy; which has been estimated at 60 cases per 100 000 pregnancies. Some epidemiological studies have reported a greater risk of VTE for women using combined oral contraceptives containing desogestrel or gestodene (the so-called third generation pills) than for women using pills containing levonorgestrel (LNG) — the so-called second generation pills' [sic: category also includes norethisterone (NET) pills]. 'The spontaneous incidence of VTE in healthy non-pregnant women (not

taking any oral contraceptive) is about 5 cases per 100 000 women per year. The incidence in users of second generation pills is about 15 per 100 000 women per year of use. The incidence in users of third generation pills is about 25 cases per 100 000 women per year of use: this excess incidence has not been satisfactorily explained by bias or confounding. *The level of all of these risks of VTE increases with age and is likely to be increased in women with other known risk factors for VTE such as obesity.*

Women must be fully informed of these very small risks ... Provided they are, the type of pill is for the woman together with her doctor or other family planning professionals jointly to decide in the light of her individual medical history. *[My emphasis.]*

The non-italicized parts of the statement, including the levels of the absolute rates of VTE, are still disputed by some authorities, and by the manufacturers of DSG and GSD products. Bias and confounding have clearly existed in the positive VTE studies; the debate is whether they explain all or only part of the difference between types of products. Even if the whole difference is accepted as real, however:

Using the rates given and assuming an estimated 1–2% mortality for VTE, there is only a 1–2 per million difference in annual VTE mortality between DSG/GSD products and LNG/NET products. This difference, from Figure 6, equates to choosing, on one Sunday afternoon in a whole year, to risk a 2-hour drive in the country rather than sitting in one's garden!

In short, autonomy in a woman's choice now has impeccable scientific and regulatory support.

Prescribing guidelines

Which women? (best for the pill method)
'Current scientific evidence suggests only two prerequisites for the safe provision of COCs: a careful personal and

family history with particular attention to cardiovascular risk factors, and a well-taken blood pressure.' [Hannaford P, Webb A. Evidence-guided prescribing of combined oral contraceptives: consensus statement. *Contraception* 1996;**54**:125–9.] Therefore:

1. Prescribers should always take a comprehensive personal and family history to exclude **absolute and relative contraindications** to the use of COCs (see Boxes on pp. 33–36). A personal history of definite VTE remains an absolute contraindication to any COC containing EE combined with any progestogen.

2. The risk factors for VTE and arterial wall disease must be assessed, separately and most carefully (see Tables 5 and 6). Alone, one risk factor from either Table is a

Table 5
Risk factors for venous thromboembolism.

Risk factor	Absolute contraindication	Relative contraindication
Family history (parent or sibling under 45)	Clotting abnormality or tests not done	Clotting factors done, normal
Overweight (high body mass index)	BMI > 39	BMI 30–39
Immobility	Confined to bed	Wheelchair life
Varicose veins (VVs)	Past thrombosis in VVs	Extensive VVs

Notes:
1. A single risk factor in relative contraindication column indicates use of LNG/NET pill, if any COC used
2. Synergism: more than one factor in the relative contraindication column means COC method is absolutely contraindicated; *also true if definite risk factor is combined with age >35*
3. The literature on the association of smoking with *venous* thromboembolic disease is mostly but not entirely negative
4. There are also important *acute* VTE risk factors which need to be considered in individual cases: notably long-haul aeroplane flights and dehydration through any cause, also recent scuba diving

Table 6
Risk factors for arterial cardiovascular system disease.

Risk factor	Absolute contraindication	Relative contraindication	Remarks
Family history of arterial CVS disease in parent or sibling <45	Known atherogenic lipid profile – or tests not available	Acceptable blood lipid profile or first attack in relative >45	POP is usually a better choice oral method for all relative contraindications + consider LNG-IUS
Cigarette smoking	? 40+ cigarettes/day	5–40 cigarettes/day	
Diabetes mellitus (DM)	Severe, or diabetic complications present (e.g. retinopathy, renal damage)	Not severe/labile, and no complications, young patient with short duration of DM	
Hypertension	BP >160/100 mmHg on repeated testing	BP 140–159/90–99 mmHg	In UK practice BP >160/95 mmHg is seen as WHO 4 (p.7)
Overweight	BMI >39	BMI 30–39	
Migraine	Focal aura symptoms; severe, or ergotamine treated	Migraine without focal aura, sumatriptan treatment	Relates to thrombotic stroke risk – see pp. 44–46 and Figure 8. If headaches without focal aura mainly in the pill-free interval, consider tricycling

Notes:

1. Synergism: if more than one relative contraindication applies, *or if woman now above aged 35, do not use COC*
2. Smoking: the risk at a given age among smokers is not reached until 10 years later by non-smokers, implying that smoking 'ages the arteries'
3. Note overweight appears in both Tables 5 and 6 – if that is the sole risk factor it indicates use of a LNG/NET pill (i.e. Table 5 takes precedence). Best choices: Loestrin 20 or the new 20 µg EE+LNG pill
4. Some of the numbers selected are arbitrary and perhaps too strict if they are the sole problem (for example the COC might actually be allowed, reluctantly, to a currently healthy 25-year-old admitting to two packs of cigarettes a day). They also relate to use for contraception. Use of COCs for medical indications often entails a different risk/benefit analysis — i.e. the extra therapeutic benefits may outweigh expected extra risks.

relative contraindication (second column of each Table) unless it is particularly severe (first column). Multiple risk factors, or any one arterial or venous factor in the Tables, when combined with age above 35 years, always have the same significance: with few exceptions, *the COC should be avoided* (**absolutely contraindicated**). The remarks and footnotes in these Tables are fundamental to pill prescribing.

Hereditary predispositions to VTE (thrombophilias)

Blanket screening by any blood test is not justifiable — not only would the cost be prohibitive, but there are also just too many false negatives and false positives for the occurrence of actual disease events. Almost the only indication for screening is a strong family history of one or more siblings or parents having had a VTE under age 45. This justifies testing for the genetic predispositions, including Factor V Leiden (the genetic cause of activated protein C resistance). Even if all the results are normal, the COC remains **relatively contraindicated**. The woman cannot be totally reassured, since by no means all the predisposing abnormalities of the complex haemostatic system have yet been characterized. Like all with one VTE-linked relative contraindication (3rd column of Table 5), such a woman should receive a LNG/NET pill — at least, unless there is a *therapeutic indication* (see important footnote 4 to Table 6).

Acquired predispositions (thrombophilias)

Antiphospholipid antibodies which increase both VTE and arterial disease risk may appear in a number of connective tissue disorders, and if identified they absolutely contraindicate the COC.

Which pill? (current 'best buys' for women)

1. First, all marketed pills may now be considered 'first line' (see bold section in DoH statement above). Given the tiny possible difference in VTE mortality between the two 'generations', the woman's own choice of a DSG or

GSD product after (well-documented) discussion must be respected: even if based on no more than the presence of acne, a friend's recommendation or the need for better cycle control, or indeed her perception of any issue of quality of life — either initially or if side effects (pp. 40–41) appear with a LNG or NET product at any later stage. 'The informed user should be the chooser.'

2. Young first-time users: despite what has just been said, a low-dose LNG or NET product should in my view remain the *usual* first choice. This is because they will include an unknown subgroup who are VTE-predisposed, VTE being a more relevant consideration than arterial disease at this age, and the pills are cheaper.

3. In the presence of a single risk factor for venous thrombosis: the new SPCs (data sheets) for COCs state that DSG/GSD products are contraindicated (WHO 4). I would agree that a LNG or NET product is certainly preferred, if COC is used at all **for contraception**. If used for **therapy**, a different risk/benefit balance may apply: e.g. a woman with a BMI of 31 who because of having severe acne with or without polycystic ovarian disease needs Marvelon or Dianette (the latter in my view shares the same oestrogen-dominant category).

4. Women with a single definite arterial risk factor, usually after a number of years' VTE-free use, *or* if COC is used at all by a healthy and risk factor free woman above age 35: changing to a DSG or GSD product might be (at least) discussed. Any advantages in so doing are far from established (pp. 23, 25); *the primary reason for changing brands is the control of side effects.*

In premenopausal women AMI is almost exclusively a disease of *smokers*. No study, and there have been at least five good ones (RCGP, Oxford/FPA, US Nurses, WHO and MICA, 1999), has been able to detect an increased risk of AMI either in current or past pill-taking *non-smokers*. The available evidence is similar for thrombotic and haemorrhagic strokes. So the arterial event risk of using **all** the modern low-oestrogen brands must be very small if not absent for women free of arterial risk factors. However, the risk is high when arterial risk factors are present (the RCGP's relative risk estimate for AMI was 20.8 for smoking pill-takers) and increases with age. Moreover the case-fatality rate for AMI in pill-takers is also much higher. Thus, I feel that we should not discount the suggestive indirect evidence that DSG/GSD pills might have relative advantages for arterial wall disease, *but only in higher risk women*.

Therefore, switching to a low oestrogen DSG or GSD pill may reasonably be discussed with women who have any significant arterial risk factor *as they get older*, for two reasons:

- It is only in the older age group that arterial disease becomes common enough to be relevant to prescribing policy
- Any woman who has by then been for some years on any combined pill — EE combined with any progestogen — and/or has had a full-term pregnancy, is a 'survivor': relatively unlikely now to get VTE (not that this previous uncomplicated use eliminates that risk)

Femodette (GSD) or Mercilon (DSG) are the 20 μg EE products which are my own usual suggestion for these women (*no later than age 35*) and for arterial risk factor-free women aged 35–50. Loestrin 20 or the new 20 mg EE+LNG pill when available would also be acceptable — and better if there is any special concern about venous (VTE) risk.

Documentation
If a DSG/GSD pill is chosen, whether for this indication or more often just because the woman prefers it on quality of life or side effect grounds, there must be a full contemporaneous record:

- Of the risk factor history
- That the woman accepts a possibly increased risk of VTE relative to other formulations

---

Norgestimate, the progestogen in Cilest

Initially there were no good epidemiological data, so the CSM letter in 1995 left prescribing practice unchanged for this product. It is a fact that 20% of norgestimate ingested actually becomes LNG, by metabolism. Thus, all Cilest users actually finish up with a pill which effectively delivers 55 µg of LNG. This, if the above thinking is correct, may provide some counteraction of the oestrogenicity (and pro-thrombogenicity) of the EE in Cilest.

In practice, we can continue to use Cilest without the concerns generated by the CSM letter of 18 October 1995. Pending more data, Cilest seems to be working out as a slightly oestrogen-dominant 'middle of the road' compound, useful for *many* women, but not especially for when one has a specific concern either about VTE or about the arterial walls.

Absolute contraindications to COCs

These are WHO 4. However, progestogen-only pills (POPs) and other progestogen-only methods are often only WHO 2 at most.

COCs — all brands — are absolutely contraindicated in:

A. Past or present circulatory disease
- Any past proven arterial or venous thrombosis
- Ischaemic heart disease or angina, Kawasaki disease (WHO 3 after full recovery)
- Severe or combined risk factors for venous or arterial disease (see Tables 5 and 6)
- Atherogenic lipid disorders (take advice from expert, as indicated)
- Known prothrombotic abnormality of coagulation/fibrinolysis, i.e. congenital or acquired thrombophilias (p. 30); from at least 2 (preferably 4) weeks before until 2 weeks after mobilization following elective major or leg surgery (do not demand that the COC be stopped for minor surgery such as laparoscopy); during leg immobilization (e.g. after fracture or varicose vein treatment); and during short-term exposure to high altitude (above 4500 m: lower heights are WHO 3)

- Migraines with the features described on p. 44
- Transient ischaemic attacks even without headache
- Past cerebral haemorrhage, which can be secondary to cerebral venous thrombosis (also to avoid COC-related rise in blood pressure if past subarachnoid bleed)
- Most types of structural heart disease (must discuss with cardiologist): atrial fibrillation, atrial septal defect (risk of paradoxical embolism), pulmonary hypertension

B. Disease of the liver
- Active liver disease (whenever liver function tests currently abnormal, including infiltrations and cirrhosis); recurrent or pill-related cholestatic jaundice or cholestatic jaundice in pregnancy (history of mild case can be WHO 3); Dubin–Johnson and Rotor syndromes (Gilbert's disease is WHO 2). Following viral hepatitis COCs may be resumed 3 months after liver function tests have become normal
- Liver adenoma, carcinoma
- Gallstones (but COCs may be used after cholecystectomy)
- The acute hepatic porphyrias; others are usually WHO 3, but non-steroid hormone method usually preferable (see also p. 65.)

C. History of serious condition affected by sex steroids or related to previous COC use
- Systemic lupus erythematosus (SLE) — also VTE risk
- COC-induced hypertension
- Pancreatitis due to hypertriglyceridaemia
- Pemphigoid gestationis
- Chorea
- Stevens–Johnson syndrome (erythema multiforme), if COC-associated
- Trophoblastic disease but only until hCG levels are undetectable*

D. Pregnancy

E. Undiagnosed genital tract bleeding

F. Oestrogen-dependent neoplasms
- Breast cancer (some oncologists permit COCs in selected cases in prolonged remission)
- Past breast biopsy showing premalignant epithelial atypia

G. Miscellaneous
- Allergy to any pill constituent
- Haemolytic uraemic syndrome
- Past benign intracranial hypertension

H. Woman's anxiety about COC safety unrelieved by counselling

---

* In the USA this is not considered a contraindication while hCG is present, partly because chemotherapy is given to almost all cases of trophoblastic disease, thereby obliterating any hormonal effect

Note that several of the above (e.g. D, E, F, H) are not necessarily permanent contraindications. Over the years many women have been unnecessarily deprived of COCs for reasons now shown to have no link, such as thrush, or which would have positively benefited from the method, such as secondary amenorrhoea with hypo-oestrogenism. Indeed, the COC can be a good choice if that occurs in long-term users of an injectable (see pp. 70–71) — unless the COC is itself contraindicated.

Relative contraindications to COCs

The Box below lists the relative contraindications, signifying that the COC method is usable in context with:

- The benefit–risk evaluation for that individual
- The acceptability or otherwise of alternatives
- Sometimes with special advice (e.g. in migraine, to report a change of symptomatology) or monitoring

In cases with excess risk of venous thrombosis, if the pill is used at all for contraception it should be a LNG/NET variety.

Relative contraindications to COCs (WHO 2 unless otherwise stated):
- Risk factors for arterial or venous disease (Tables 5 and 6). These are usually WHO 3, provided normally that only one is present, and not to a marked degree
- Homozygous sickle cell disease (see p. 37)
- Long-term partial immobilization — e.g. in a wheelchair (use LNG/NET pill)
- Sex steroid-dependent cancer in remission. (Melanoma is WHO 2 for the pill)
- Oligo-/amenorrhoea (COCs may be prescribed after investigation — may even be WHO 1 — to supply oestrogen in a woman needing contraception or to control the symptoms of polycystic ovary syndrome)
- Hyperprolactinaemia (relative contraindication WHO 3 for patients under specialist supervision)

- Very severe depression, if likely to be exacerbated by COCs (but unwanted pregnancies can be very depressing)
- Some chronic diseases: inflammatory bowel disease, which produces prothrombotic changes especially in exacerbations, including severe Crohn's disease (WHO 3 or WHO 4 for the variety which can be brought on by COCs); diabetes (WHO 3 but can be 4, see Table 6 and below); essential hypertension, well-controlled; otosclerosis (some authorities permit supervised COC use; WHO 3)
- Diseases that require long-term treatment with drugs which might interact with COCs (see pp. 52–56) — WHO 2

Weak relative contraindications:
- If a young first-degree relation has breast cancer
- Established benign breast disease (without atypia, p. 14)

Intercurrent diseases

It is impossible for the Boxes to list every known disease which might have a bearing (i.e. WHO 4, 3 or 2) on COC prescription, and for many the data are unavailable. A working rule therefore is to ascertain whether or not the condition might lead to **summation** with known major adverse effects of COCs, particularly with the risk of any circulatory disease; this usually means WHO 4. If it won't, in most serious chronic conditions the patient can be reassured that COCs are not known to have any effect, good or bad; they should then be used (WHO 2), though with the most careful monitoring and alertness for the onset of new risk factors. Reliable protection from pregnancy is often particularly important when other diseases are present.

The LNG IUS (pp. 94–99) has very few contraindications and is therefore becoming the first choice hormonal method in many chronic disease states

Diabetes (generally WHO 3)
Mercilon or Femodette (see p. 32) can be valuable for limited periods, under careful supervision and provided that

there is no arteriopathy, retinopathy, neuropathy or renal damage (or obesity or smoking!), and preferably if the duration of the diabetes has been short (Table 6). The POP or Implanon are good alternative options, with perhaps a modern copper IUD, the LNG IUS or sterilization to follow later.

Hypertension
Hypertension is an important risk factor for heart disease and stroke. In most women on COCs there is a slight increase in both systolic and diastolic blood pressure within the normotensive range. Approximately 1% become clinically hypertensive (WHO 4 for the pill, if clearly pill-induced) and the rate increases with age and duration of use. Past pregnancy-induced hypertension does not predispose to hypertension during COC use but it is a risk factor for myocardial infarction, very markedly so if the women also smokes, and is then WHO 3. See also pp. 29, 42.

Sickle cell disorders
Sickle cell *trait* has no bearing on COCs. Both homozygous sickle cell disease and COCs individually lead to an increased risk of thrombosis, superimposed during the arterial stasis of a crisis. Hence most manufacturers have for many years included frank sickling diseases among the absolute contraindications to COCs. However, a review of studies in West Africa and the West Indies suggests that sickle cell disease is only a weak relative contraindication (WHO 2), especially when balanced against the particularly serious risks of pregnancy. In the UK injectables or the LNG IUS are normally better choices.

Second choice of pill brand

Some women react unpredictably, and it is a false expectation that any single pill will suit all women. Individual variations in motivation and tolerance of minor side effects are well recognized. But, due to differences in absorption and metabolism there is also marked variability (threefold, in the

Figure 7
Schematic representation of the marked individual variation in blood levels of both contraceptive steroids and rationale of suggested 'titration'.

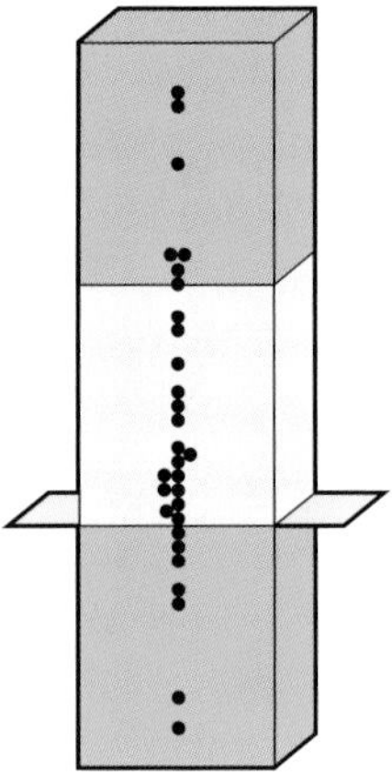

Zone of high blood levels
(? ↑Metabolic impact)
(? ↑More non-bleeding side effects)

'Ideal' zone

Bleeding threshold

Zone of breakthrough bleeding

area under the curve) in *blood levels of the exogenous hormones* (Figure 7).

Breakthrough bleeding

Prescribers should try to identify the lowest dose for each woman which does not cause breakthrough bleeding (BTB). This should minimize adverse side effects, both serious and minor, and also reduce measurable metabolic changes. Since combined pills all have a powerful contraceptive effect, this approach does not impair effectiveness (far more important is not lengthening the pill-free interval, see pp. 48–49). Indeed, even if BTB occurs, extra contraception (e.g. with condoms) does not need to be advised — provided there is ongoing good compliance with pill-taking.

The objective is that each woman should receive the least long-term metabolic impact that her uterus will allow — i.e. the lowest dose of contraceptive steroids that is just, but only just, above her bleeding threshold. If there is good cycle control, therefore, and a lower-dose brand in the same 'ladder' (Figure 4) is available, switching to it should be considered at the time of repeat prescription.

If BTB occurs and is unacceptable or persists beyond two cycles, a different or higher dose brand (Figure 4) should be tried, subject to the checks in the Box below. Phasic COCs are second-choice formulations in my own practice, but they are certainly worth trying for BTB and especially for absence of withdrawal bleeding. Among these, Gracial (not yet available at time of writing) has a particularly good reputation for cycle control. If cycle control can only be achieved by a 50 µg oestrogen pill, this could be justifiable with good counselling, monitoring and records (but check Tables 5 and 6).

It is vital to exclude other causes of BTB before blaming the COC!

Checklist for abnormal bleeding in a pill-user

- **DISEASE** Examine the cervix (it is not unknown for bleeding from an invasive cancer to be wrongly attributed, and any bloodstained discharge should always trigger the thought '*Chlamydia?*')
- **DISORDERS of PREGNANCY** that cause bleeding (e.g. trophoblastic tumour, or retained products if COC was started after a recent termination of pregnancy)
- **DEFAULT** (BTB may start 2 or 3 days after missed pills and may be persistent thereafter)
- **DRUGS**, primarily enzyme inducers (see text). Cigarettes have also been implicated: BTB is statistically more common among smokers
- **Diarrhoea** and/or **VOMITING** (diarrhoea alone has to be very severe to impair absorption significantly)
- **DISTURBANCES of ABSORPTION**, for example after massive gut resection (coeliac disease does not pose an absorption problem)
- **Diet** (the gut flora involved in recycling ethinyloestradiol may be reduced in vegetarians, but this is a very unlikely cause)
- **DURATION of USE** too short — i.e. assessment too early (minimal BTB which is tolerable may resolve after 2–3 months' use of any new formulation). The opposite possibility may apply during 'tricycling' (see pp. 51–52), namely that duration of continuous use has been too long for that woman's endometrium to be sustained: in which case 'bicycling' of two packets in a row may be substituted
- **DOSE**, after the above have been excluded, it is possible to try a phasic pill if the woman is receiving monophasic treatment; to increase the progestogen component (or oestrogen if Mercilon is in use); to try a different progestogen; or to consider a 50 µg pill (see text)

The preceding, very helpful, checklist was modified from Sapire E, *Contraception and Sexuality in Health and Disease* (New York: McGraw-Hill, 1990).

Second choice if there are non-bleeding side effects

The use of contemporary pills has reduced the reporting of so-called 'minor' side effects. When symptoms occur it is generally bad practice to give further prescriptions, such as diuretics for weight gain, antimigraine treatments or anti-depressants. For depression, however, pyridoxine up to 50 mg daily may be beneficial (if continued for at least 2 months).

Otherwise there are two main preferred, if empirical, courses of action: to decrease the dose of either hormone, if still possible (in the limit, oestrogen can be eliminated by a trial of the POP); or to change to a different progestogen. Although the evidence is mainly anecdotal, there is some more specific guidance available for side effects and conditions associated with a relative excess of either steroid.

Which second choice of pill? Relative oestrogen excess	
Symptoms	**Conditions**
• Nausea	• Benign breast disease
• Dizziness	• Fibroids
• 'Premenstrual tension' and irritability	• Endometriosis
• Cyclical weight gain (fluid), 'bloating'	
• Vaginal discharge (no infection)	
• Some cases of breast enlargement/pain	

Treat with progestogen-dominant COC, such as Microgynon 30, Loestrin 30, Eugynon 30 (but with caution regarding lipids, and risk of arterial disease in those with the relevant risk factors, see pp. 29, 31–32). Loestrin 20 and the new 20 mg EE+LNG pill are oestrogen-deficient options

Symptoms	Conditions

• Dryness of vagina
• Some cases of:
  Sustained weight gain
  Depression
  Loss of libido
  Lassitude
  Breast symptoms (other)
	• Acne/seborrhoea
	• Hirsutism

Treat with oestrogen-dominant COC, such as Ovysmen/Brevinor, or Marvelon; Gracial, when it becomes available; then Dianette (see text). (Caution necessary in that oestrogen dominance may correlate with a slightly higher risk of venous thrombosis, especially if relevant risk factors present, see pp. 28, 30–32)

More about Dianette

This is an anti-androgen plus oestrogen combination (cyproterone acetate [CPA] 2 mg with EE 35 µg), for the treatment of moderately severe acne and mild hirsutism in women. These are its indications, but it is also a reliable anovulant like other COCs, and has similar rules for missed tablets, interactions, absolute and relative contraindications, and requirements for monitoring.

Although practically everything about the COC applies also to Dianette, it is an oestrogen-dominant product. As it permits EE to raise SHBG and HDL-cholesterol, it might potentially also allow the oestrogen to have relatively greater effects in a prothrombotic direction than a LNG product would (see pp. 22–23 above). There are no clear epidemiological data, but the current working hypothesis is to put it in a similar category to a 'third generation' DSG/GSD product and follow the prescribing guidelines on pp. 27–33 yet *without* the special medico-legal considerations which were triggered by the CSM letter (pp. 22, 32).

Duration of treatment with Dianette needs to be individualized. In the Data Sheet it is recommended that 'treatment is withdrawn when the acne or hirsutism is completely resolved', but 'repeat courses may be given if the condition recurs'. There are some concerns (unconfirmed) related to hepatic effects, including benign and malignant liver tumour risk in long-term use. It is usual to encourage patients to switch (commonly to Marvelon, or perhaps Gracial) when their condition is controlled, usually after 1–3 years; if their condition relapses, it may be appropriate to use Dianette for much longer (see Table 6, p. 29, footnote 4).

Counselling, supervision and monitoring

Each woman needs individual teaching, backed by the FPA's user-friendly *Choosing and Using the Combined Pill*, which includes an important Box (similar to p. 47) listing the symptoms which should trigger taking urgent medical advice. This booklet should always be given and its publication date noted in the patient's case notes. At the MPC it is also policy to check with all follow-up patients if they still have it. Table 7 gives the recommended starting routines. After dealing with the patient's concerns about risks, benefits and 'minor' side effects, the main take-home messages to be conveyed to a new user are highlighted on p. 59.

Blood pressure
Monitoring of blood pressure is vital. It should be recorded before COCs are started and checked after 3 months (1 month in a high-risk case) and subsequently at intervals of 6 months. After about 2 years (some would say earlier) the interval can reasonably be increased to 1 year in women without risk factors, providing there is no rise between successive measurements. COCs should always be stopped altogether if blood pressure exceeds 160/100 mmHg (or more usually in the UK >160/95 mmHg, p. 29) on repeated measurements. A more moderate increase still suggests the possibility of an increased risk of arterial disease, especially in the presence of another arterial risk factor.

Table 7
Starting routines for combined oral contraceptives.

Conditions before start	Start when?	Extra precautions for 7 days
1 Menstruating	On day 1 or 2 of period	No*
	On day 3 or later	Yes*
2 Postpartum		
(a) No lactation	Day 21§ (low risk of thrombosis: first ovulations reported after day 28)	No
(b) Lactation	Not normally recommended (POP or injectable preferred)	
3 After induced abortion/miscarriage	Same day or day 2	No
4 After trophoblastic tumour	Day 21 if beyond 24 weeks One month after no hCG detected	As (1)
5 After higher dose COC	Instant switch†	No
6 After lower- or same-dose COC	After usual 7-day break	No
7 After POP	First day of period	No*
8 During POP-induced secondary amenorrhoea	Any day (end of packet)	No
9 Other secondary amenorrhoea (pregnancy excluded)‡	Any day	Yes
10 First period after postcoital contraception	By day 2 when woman sure her flow is normal	No*

*Except some 28-day (ED) pills, where extra precautions recommended for 14 days. In the other situations here, start with the first *active* tablet
§Puerperal risk lasts longer after *severe* pregnancy-related hypertension, or the related HELLP (hypertension, elevated liver enzymes, low platelets) syndrome, so delay COC use until the return of normal BP and biochemistry. This history in the past is WHO 1
†If usual 7-day break, rebound ovulation may occur at the time of transfer
‡Meaning prescriber is confident that no blastocyst or sperm is already in the upper genital tract, if necessary through a negative sensitive pregnancy test after at least 14 days of safe contraception or abstinence from intercourse

Migraine: absolute contraindications (to commencing or continuing the COC):

1. *Migraine with aura during which there are focal neurological symptoms* (usually asymmetrical and typically preceding the headache itself). The significant associated symptoms during an aura are:

- Loss of sight, or of part or whole of the field of vision on one side (homonymous visual disturbance). Teichopsia is one variety, in which a bright scintillating angulated line surrounds the area of lost vision (bright scotoma)
- Numbness, severe paraesthesia or weakness on one side of the body (e.g. one limb, side of the tongue)
- Disturbance of speech (nominal dysphasia)

Note the absence of photophobia or symmetrical blurring or mere 'flashing lights': the main feature the relevant symptoms share is that they are 'focal' or interpretable as due to (transient) cerebral ischaemia Should they occur, the artificial oestrogen of the COC should normally be stopped and thereafter avoided to minimize the risk of superimposed thrombosis causing permanent ischaemia — i.e. a thrombotic stroke

2. *Migraines that are unusually frequent/severe.* 'Status migrainosus' describes attacks lasting more than 72 hours, which contraindicate the COC absolutely — unless they resolve completely after treatment for medication misuse

3. *Migraines treated with ergot derivatives*, due to their vasoconstrictor actions

4. *Definite migraines without aura* **plus** one or more arterial risk factors — may be WHO 4 or 3 — see Figure 8 for details

   NB *Age above 35 counts as a risk factor*, and as usual any very substantial single arterial risk factor from Table 6 would be WHO 4 anyway. Using data from Denmark, the background annual risk of thrombotic stroke for women at age 20 is 2 in 100 000. With migraines more than once per month plus taking COC this rises to 10 in 100 000. But at age 40, background risk is 20 in 100 000, rising to 56 in migraine-sufferers (same attack frequency) and, with the same risk ratio (1.8) as for younger women, adding the COC makes an unacceptable 100 in 100 000 total incidence. And that is without adding the extra risk factor of focal aura

NB: in all the above any of the progestogen-only, oestrogen-free hormonal methods may be offered, immediately. Similar headaches may continue, but now without the potential added risk from prothrombotic effects of the EE. Particularly useful choices are the POP, depot medroxyprogesterone acetate (DMPA) and the LNG IUS

Migraine

Studies have shown an increased risk of ischaemic stroke in migraine sufferers and in COC users. There is good evidence of exacerbation by arterial risk factors, including increasing age above 35, and some evidence that certain features of the headaches themselves tend to focus the risk of this rare catastrophe in a pill-user. See Figure 8 and the Boxes for details. Migraines are here defined as episodic headaches with nausea and photophobia, usually one-sided, lasting 4–72 hours.

Migraine: relative contraindications

This means that the COC may be used, but always with specific instruction to the woman regarding those changes in the character or severity of her headache symptoms which mean she should stop the method and take urgent medical advice. These are in fact listed as the first six items in the Box on p. 47.

1. *Migraine without focal aura*, not in any of the categories opposite, under age 35. If these or other 'ordinary' headaches occur particularly in the pill-free interval, tricycling the COC may help (see p. 51)
2. *Distant past history during adolescence of migraine with focal aura*, before commencing the COC; the COC may be given a trial with the caveats above
3. *Occurrence of a woman's first-ever attack of migraine of any type while on the COC*. This should be stopped if she is seen during the attack, but can be later restarted with the usual forewarning about focal symptoms (and instructions to switch to another method if they occur)
4. *Use of a triptan (e.g. sumatriptan)* with no other contraindicating factors

---

Stopping COCs

The first menstruation after stopping COCs (for any reason) is often delayed. Secondary amenorrhoea for 6 months should always be investigated, whether or not it occurs after stopping COCs — the link is coincidental and not causal. Whatever the diagnosis, if there is oestrogen deficiency it should always be treated, either by hormone replacement therapy (HRT) or, if contraception is a requirement, by the COC.

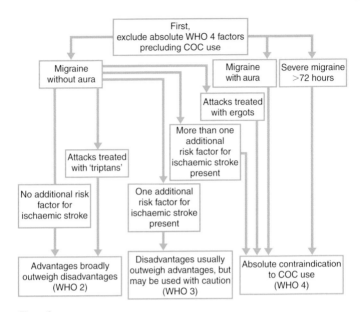

Figure 8
Flow diagram for COC use and migraine. (Reproduced from MacGregor A, Guillebaud J (1998) Br J Family Planning 24: 53–60.)

The Box on p. 47 lists the (only) reasons for discontinuing COCs immediately or soon, that should be understood by all well-counselled women from their first visit. The worst implications of most of these are pill-related thrombotic or embolic catastrophes in the making, but more often there is another explanation. They mean the EE should be stopped, but any POP method could be started immediately pending the diagnosis. They appear in lay terms in the FPA's recommended leaflet *Choosing and Using the Combined Pill*, which is one good reason why at the MPC it is policy to ensure this leaflet is made available to all users (see p. 2).

COCs should be stopped immediately, pending investigation and treatment, if the following occur:
1. Unusual or severe and very prolonged headache
2. Loss of sight in one eye, or of part or whole of the field of vision on one side
3. Disturbance of speech (nominal dysphasia)
4. Numbness, severe paraesthesia or weakness on one side of the body (e.g. one limb, side of the tongue); indeed any symptom suggesting cerebral ischaemia
5. A severe unexplained fainting attack or severe acute vertigo or ataxia
6. Focal epilepsy
7. Painful swelling in the calf
8. Pain in the chest, especially pleuritic pain
9. Breathlessness or cough with bloodstained sputum
10. Severe abdominal pain
11. Immobilization, as after sudden orthopaedic injury or *major* surgery or leg surgery: stop COC and consider heparin treatment. If elective procedure and pill stopped more than 2 weeks ahead, anticoagulation often unnecessary

Other reasons for early discontinuation:
12. Acute jaundice
13. Blood pressure above 160/100 mmHg on repeated measurement
14. Severe skin rash (e.g. erythema multiforme)
15. Detection of a new risk factor, e.g. onset of diabetes or SLE, diagnosis of a structural heart lesion such as atrial septal defect (ASD), detection of breast cancer

The 'pill-free interval' (PFI)

As no contraceptive is being taken during the PFI, it has considerable efficacy implications (Figure 9). Biochemical and ultrasound data obtained at the MPC and elsewhere demonstrate return of significant pituitary and ovarian follicular activity during the PFI in about one-fifth of cases — to a marked extent in some. Therefore, breakthrough ovulation is likely to follow any lengthening of the PFI. Figure 9 is a useful representation since the horseshoe is a symmetrical object. Lengthening of the PFI might be caused 'either side of the horseshoe' — i.e. from omissions, malabsorption as from vomiting, or drug interactions involving pills either at the start or at the end of a packet.

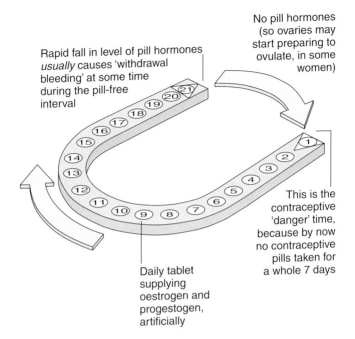

No pill hormones (so ovaries may start preparing to ovulate, in some women)

Rapid fall in level of pill hormones *usually* causes 'withdrawal bleeding' at some time during the pill-free interval

This is the contraceptive 'danger' time, because by now no contraceptive pills taken for a whole 7 days

Daily tablet supplying oestrogen and progestogen, artificially

Figure 9
'Horseshoe' analogy to explain the 21-day cycle.

Thus the former advice to the woman who has missed pills — to take extra precautions to the end of her packet or the next withdrawal bleed — is wrong, as it fails to allow for the return of ovarian activity in the PFI.

In 1986, a population of current pill-users was studied after the end of a routine PFI. The study showed that if only 14 or even as few as 7 pills were then taken, no ovulation occurred after 7 pills were subsequently missed. This implies at the very least that up to 4 pills may be missed mid-packet with impunity (see p. 105). This and other work may be summarized as follows:

- 7 consecutive pills are enough 'to shut the door on the ovaries' (therefore pills 8–21, or longer during tricycling, simply 'keep the door shut')
- 7 pills can be omitted without ovulation, as indeed is regularly the case in the pill-free week
- More than 7 pills missed (*in total*) risks ovulation

The '**7-day advice**' as used by the FPA is based on this pharmacology (Figure 10). If 28-day packs are used, which help to avoid risky 'late restarts', the user must learn which are the dummy 'reminder' tablets. These must be omitted to avoid an added routine break if she makes her own break prematurely — through missing some of the last 7 active pills. All women should be asked to report back if they have no bleeding in the *next* PFI.

Vomiting and diarrhoea

Extra contraceptive precautions should start from the onset of illness and continue for 7 days after it ends, with elimination of the pill-free interval as indicated above. If vomiting began over 2 hours after one pill was taken, it can be assumed to have been absorbed. Diarrhoea alone is not a problem, unless it is of cholera-like severity.

Previous combined pill failure

Women who have had a previous COC failure may claim perfect compliance or perhaps admit to omission of no more than 1 pill. Either way, as surveys show that most women miss a tablet quite frequently but very few conceive, the ability to do so probably tells us more about the individual's physiology than her memory. She is likely to be a member of that one-fifth of the population whose ovaries show above average return to activity in the PFI. It is therefore recommended that such women be advised to take three packets in a row (the tricycle regimen, see Figure 11) followed by a shortened PFI. Six days is often a good choice for the PFI as it is easy to remember, the start day of each tricycle being identical to the weekday it finished (and can

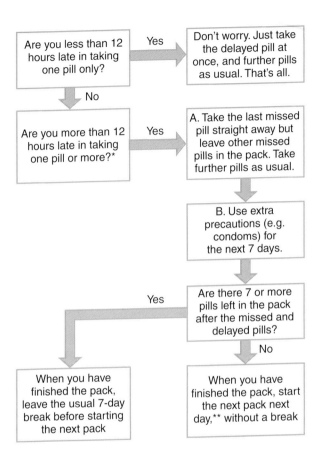

| Are you less than 12 hours late in taking one pill only? | **Yes** → | Don't worry. Just take the delayed pill at once, and further pills as usual. That's all. |

↓ No

| Are you more than 12 hours late in taking one pill or more?* | **Yes** → | A. Take the last missed pill straight away but leave other missed pills in the pack. Take further pills as usual. |

B. Use extra precautions (e.g. condoms) for the next 7 days.

Are there 7 or more pills left in the pack after the missed and delayed pills?

Yes ← | → **No**

When you have finished the pack, leave the usual 7-day break before starting the next pack

When you have finished the pack, start the next pack next day,** without a break

Figure 10
Advice for missed pills (21-day packaging).
If two or more pills missed **and if they were all from the first seven in your pack, and if you have had unprotected intercourse since the end of your last pack, talk promptly to your doctor. You may need emergency pills **as well as** continuing with instructions A and B above. See p. 105.*
**Even with triphasic pills, you should go straight to (the first phase of) the same brand. You may bleed a bit but you will still strengthen your contraception. This is quite different from postponing a 'period'. See p. 51.

also be used to 'strengthen' contraceptively any 20 µg pill such as Loestrin 20). The gap may be shortened further in high-risk cases, such as during the use of enzyme inducers (see pp. 53–55).

Once it has been appreciated that the 'Achilles heel' of the COC is the PFI, the COC can always be made 'stronger' as a contraceptive, by eliminating and/or shortening the PFI through variations on the tricycling theme depicted in Figure 11. See also 'bicycling', below.

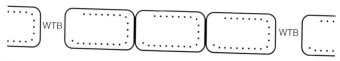

Figure 11
Tricycling (three packs in a row). Note that they must be monophasic packs. Duration of PFI may also be shortened. WTB = withdrawal bleeds.

Why have pill-free intervals at all?
The pill-free week does promote a reassuring withdrawal bleed and, indeed, if this does not occur in two successive cycles it is best to eliminate pregnancy using a sensitive urine test. However, its importance could be greater in that it may allow some recovery from systemic effects. In a study of medium-dose LNG-containing pills, HDL-cholesterol suppression was eliminated by the end of the PFI. Hence it is probably wise to omit the gap between packets only in the short term (upon request) to avoid a 'period' on special occasions*; or, longer term, for special indications as listed in the Box below, using the tricycle regimen. This leads to only about five withdrawal bleeds and, for the first listed indication, only five withdrawal headaches per year.

---

* Users of phasic pills who wish to postpone withdrawal bleeds must use the final phase of a spare packet, or pills from an equivalent formulation, e.g. Norimin in the case of Trinovum, or Microgynon immediately after the last tablet of Logynon.

BTB (p. 39) may occur during tricycling, as a result of that pill in that woman being unable to maintain endometrial stability for so long. The solution may then be to 'bicycle' (42 days of continuous pill-taking) followed, depending on the indication, by a shortened pill-free gap.

Indications for the tricycling regimen shown in Figure 8, using a monophasic pill

- Headaches, including migraine without aura, and other bothersome symptoms if they occur regularly in the withdrawal week
- Unacceptably heavy or painful withdrawal bleeds
- Paradoxically, to help women who are concerned about absent withdrawal bleeds (less frequent pregnancy tests for reassurance)
- Premenstrual syndrome — tricycling helps when COCs are used (p. 9)
- Epilepsy, which benefits from relatively more sustained levels of the administered hormones, and tricycling may also be indicated by the therapy given
- Enzyme-inducer therapy (see text)
- Endometriosis, where a progestogen-dominant monophasic pill may be tricycled for maintenance treatment after primary therapy
- Wherever there is suspicion of decreased efficacy (see text)
- At the woman's choice

Drug interactions

Drug interactions reduce the efficacy of COCs mainly by induction of liver enzymes, which leads to increased elimination of both oestrogen and progestogen (Figure 12). Additionally, in a very small (but unknown) minority of women, disturbance by certain broad-spectrum antibiotics of the gut flora which normally split oestrogen metabolites that arrive in the bowel can reduce the reabsorption of reactivated oestrogen. This effect is not a factor in the maintenance of progestogen levels and so is irrelevant to the POP. The most clinically important drugs with which interaction occurs are:

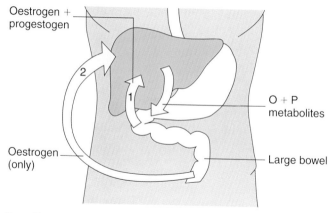

Figure 12
The enterohepatic recirculation of oestrogen.

Enzyme inducers (important examples)
- Rifampicin, rifabutin
- Griseofulvin (antifungal)
- Barbiturates
- Phenytoin
- Carbamazepine
- Primidone
- Topiramate
- Modafinil
- Lansoprazole
- Some anti-retro virals (e.g. ritonavir) — take advice
- St John's Wort — potency varies; CSM advises *non-use*

Broad-spectrum antibiotics (less important)
- Ampicillin, amoxycillin and related penicillins
- Tetracyclines
- Broad-spectrum cephalosporins

Note that other older anti-epileptics (ethosuximide, valproate and clonazepam) and most newer ones (including vigabatrin and lamotrigine) do not pose this problem. Among antimicrobials, co-trimoxazole and erythromycin actually tend to raise blood levels of EE, although not dangerously.

Short-term use of any interacting drug/long-term broad-spectrum antibiotics

Extra contraceptive precautions are advised during the treatment and should then be continued for a further 7 days, with elimination of the next PFI as appropriate from Figure 10, based on when in the pill packet the last potentially less effective pill was taken. The stakes are particularly high with **griseofulvin** because of its strong teratogenicity.

Rifampicin is such a powerful enzyme inducer that even if it is given only for 2 days (for instance to eliminate carriage of the meningococcus), increased elimination by the liver must be assumed for 4 weeks thereafter. Extra contraception or a stronger pill with elimination of one or more PFIs (see below) should be recommended to cover that time.

With **broad-spectrum antibiotics** the large-bowel flora responsible for recycling oestrogens are reconstituted with resistant organisms within about 2 weeks. In practice, therefore, if COCs are commenced in a women who has been taking a tetracycline long term, there is no need to advise extra contraceptive precautions. There is a potential problem (now believed to involve very few women but clinically we never know which) only in the reverse situation — when the tetracycline is first introduced to treat a long-term COC-user. Even then, extra precautions need only be sustained for 14 days plus the 'usual' 7 days, with elimination of the next PFI if the first 2 weeks of antibiotic use involved any of the last 7 pills of a pack.

Long-term use of enzyme inducers

This applies chiefly to epileptic women and women being treated for tuberculosis. An alternative method of contraception should always be discussed, such as an IUD or DMPA with a shortened (10-week) injection interval. Users of **rifampicin/rifabutin** should avoid the COC, and if DMPA is used an 8-week injection interval is safest. Otherwise, if the combined pill is chosen, it is recommended to prescribe initially a preparation containing 50 µg oestrogen, using the tricycle regimen described above. This reduces the number of contraceptively risky PFIs, and is particularly appropriate for epileptic women since the frequency of attacks is often reduced by the maintenance of steady hormone levels. The PFI should also, logically, be shortened at the end of each tricycle. At the MPC we advise that the next packet should begin after 4 days, even if the withdrawal bleed has not stopped.

Only two 50 µg pills remain on the market (Table 3), and since the metabolic conversion of the pro-drug mestranol to EE is only about 75% efficient, Norinyl-1 is almost identical to Norimin. Ovran is therefore the sole choice as a single 50 µg tablet. If this is not appropriate for any reason one may be forced to construct a 50 or 60 µg regimen from two sub-50 µg products. As this practice is unlicensed the rationale for it in the individual case must be well documented on the case card, following the criteria summarized on pp. 114–115.

BTB may be the first clue to a drug interaction and also indicates appropriate alterations to the prescription, or a change of method. If the long-term user of an enzyme inducer develops BTB, the first step — after a vaginal examination and other assessments in the checklist on p. 39 — may be to try 2 or more tablets a day, if necessary to provide a combined oestrogen content of 80, 90 or 100 µg (a rare maximum). In this way, the usual policy (p. 38) of giving the minimum dose of both hormones to finish just above the threshold for bleeding can be followed. The woman can be reassured that she is metaphorically 'climbing a down escalator' — her increased liver metabolism means that she is still in reality receiving a low-dose regimen (but see p. 114, again).

Discontinuation of enzyme inducers
It may be 4 or more weeks before the level of excretory function in the liver reverts to normal. Hence if any enzyme

inducer has been used for a month or more (or at all in the case of a rifamycin), there should be a delay of about 4 weeks before the return to a standard low-dose regimen. This period should be increased to 8 weeks after more prolonged use of enzyme inducers, and logically there should then be no gap between the higher-dose and low-dose packets.

Special considerations

Duration of use
Many important benefits are enhanced as duration of COC use increases. There need be no restriction on duration of use for healthy non-smokers up to the maximum age (see below). However, pending more data, it is prudent to restrict total accumulated duration of use to a maximum of about 15 years in all smokers and others with arterial risk factors.

Maximum age for COC use
In selected healthy migraine-free non-smokers, with modern pills and careful monitoring, the many gynaecological and other benefits of COCs are now felt to outweigh the small increased cardiovascular (and breast cancer) risk of a modern pill up to age 50. Depending on her choice, an appropriate COC (most commonly Mercilon or Femodette, see p. 32) may thus be preferable to hormone replacement therapy (HRT) up to age 50 for women who need contraception as well as a supplement to diminished ovarian function. Pending more data, smokers above age 35 who request hormonal contraception should use a progestogen-only method; an IUD or IUS or perhaps vasectomy may be even better.

Beyond 50, the age-related increased COC risks are usually unacceptable for all, since fertility is now so low that less powerful contraceptives will suffice — e.g. barriers or Delfen foam (pp. 111–112).

Most forms of HRT are not contraceptive but may of course be indicated along with a simple contraceptive, once oestrogen is no longer being supplied by the COC.

The diagnosis of loss of fertility at the menopause always requires care, and raised follicle-stimulating hormone (FSH) measurements, although more reliable above age 50, are *not* diagnostic. There are preliminary data to suggest that a raised FSH at the end of the PFI may indicate that the ovaries have ceased to function. This should be confirmed by a repeat 6 weeks off all therapy. Above 50, a second high FSH result along with vasomotor symptoms and amenorrhoea (to date and continuing) is *suggestive* of final ovarian failure. The woman should be warned that the *risk of later ovulation cannot be excluded*, but she may choose to discontinue contraception, or to use a simple contraceptive until the 'officially approved' 1 year after her last bleed that was not hormonally induced.

Another protocol, which may be more acceptable to some, is to switch at 50 to the POP. If amenorrhoea and vasomotor symptoms follow (either immediately, or months or years later), FSH measurements while still taking the POP can help to confirm ovarian failure — see page 67.

Congenital abnormalities and fertility
Any possible effect of COCs on congenital abnormalities is hard to establish because it is so difficult to prove a negative, and 2% of all full-term fetuses have a significant malformation. The conclusions of a WHO scientific group have not been challenged — namely, there is no good evidence for any adverse effects on the fetus of COCs used prior to the conception cycle. Even with exposure during organogenesis, meta-analyses of the major studies also fail to show increased risk. If present it must be very small.

It should certainly do no harm if a woman stops COCs for 2 or more months before conception, but there is no objective evidence that it is worth the effort: certainly any woman who finds herself pregnant immediately after stopping COCs should be strongly reassured. Fertile ovulation is in fact often somewhat delayed, though there is no evidence that COCs can cause permanent loss of fertility.

What about 'taking breaks'?
If a woman feels more comfortable taking a routine break from the COC, we should always help her to find a satisfactory contraceptive alternative. However, there is no known benefit either to fertility or to health from taking short elective breaks of 6 months or so every few years, as was once recommended: in one study a quarter of young women who took such breaks had unwanted conceptions. Moreover, regular PFIs give the body plenty of 'breaks' (totalling 130 every 10 years!) from the COC and these might even increase the method's safety (p. 51).

Screening
Cervical screening should be performed regularly, as recommended for all sexually active women. *Routine* breast or bimanual examinations in asymptomatic pill-takers are uncalled for, the latter because most of the disorders causing detectable pelvic masses or tenderness are, as listed on p. 9, actually less frequent in COC-takers than in the partners of condom users.

Summary
The first visit for COCs is by far the most important, and should never be rushed. Often it is useful to share it between doctor and practice nurse. Quite often one of the newer long-term 'forgettable' contraceptive choices is relevant to the discussion (see p. 3), despite the woman's presenting request for what she happens to know about (the pill). If this is still her choice, after discussing the risks and benefits and fully assessing her medical and family history, all at her level of understanding, there is still much ground to cover:

Take-home messages for a new pill-taker
1. Your FPA leaflet is not to be read and thrown away, it is something to keep safely in a drawer somewhere for ongoing reference
2. The pill only works if you take it correctly: if you do, each new pack will always start on the same day of the week
3. Even if bleeding like a 'period' occurs (breakthrough bleeding), carry on pill-taking. It will usually stop, just like other early symptoms (e.g. nausea). Feel free to ring for advice about this — or any other symptom.
4. Lovemaking during the 7 days after any packet is only safe if you do go on to the next one: otherwise (if you are going to take a break from the pill) start using condoms after the last pill in the pack
5. Even if your 'period' has not stopped yet, or for any other reason, *never start your next packet late*. This is because the pill-free time is obviously a time when your ovaries are not getting the contraceptive, so might anyway be beginning to escape from its actions. (This simple explanation should always be given, it greatly improves compliance)
6. For what to do if any pill(s) are more than 12 hours late, see p. 50
7. Other things that may stop the pill from working include vomiting and some drugs (pp. 49, 52–56)
8. See a doctor at once if the things on p. 47 occur
9. As a one-off manoeuvre you can shorten one pill-free gap to make sure your withdrawal bleeds avoid weekends

And, finally:
10. Good though it is for contraception, the pill does not give adequate protection against *Chlamydia* and other STIs. Whenever in any doubt, especially with a new partner, use a condom as well

Thereafter there are really only three key components to COC-monitoring — namely:

- Blood pressure (p. 42)
- Headaches (pp. 44–47)
- Identification and management of any new risk factors/diseases/side effects

As well as routine appointments, there must also be freedom for each woman to report back for advice at any time, maybe to the practice nurse.

In conclusion, the combined pill provides highly acceptable contraception for many. However, no matter how carefully those with contraindications are excluded, a few women will experience adverse effects. Presentation of multiple side effects may indicate the need for a different method; however, excessive anxiety should first be suspected and possible psychosexual aspects may need to be discussed.

Transdermal combined oral contraception

At the time of writing Evra, a skin patch for contraception, was at an advanced stage in the regulatory process for the countries of the European Union. Each patch delivers a combination of 17-deacetyl norgestimate, the chief active metabolite of norgestimate, and ethinyloestradiol via the skin of the abdomen or buttock over a period of seven days — both in the same therapeutic range as oral Cilest. After three patches have been used the woman takes a seven-day patch-free interval before the next cycle.

Both the effectiveness and the side effect profile of Evra appear to be very similar to Cilest, aside from the occurrence of some allergic skin reactions. This new choice of method will be welcome: it is expected to assist women who have difficulty in remembering to take a daily pill, as well as avoiding all absorption problems arising from gastrointestinal disorders or broad spectrum antibiotics.

Progestogen-only pill

There are six varieties of progestogen-only pill (POP) available (Table 8). If POPs are taken absolutely regularly each day within a timespan of a couple of hours, without breaks and regardless of bleeding patterns, they are almost as effective as COCs, especially for those aged 30 and over. In the UK the Oxford/FPA study reported a failure rate of 3.1/100 woman-years at age 25–29, but this improved to 1.0 at 35–39 years and was as low as 0.3 for women over 40 years. Efficacy is also much greater during full lactation, approaching that of COCs.

Table 8
Available progestogen-only pills.

Product	Constituents	Course of treatment
Noriday	350 µg norethisterone	28 tablets
Micronor	350 µg norethisterone	28 tablets
Femulen	500 µg ethynodiol diacetate	28 tablets
Neogest	75 µg dl norgestrel*	35 tablets
Norgeston	30 µg levonorgestrel	35 tablets
Microval	30 µg levonorgestrel	35 tablets
Cerazette§	75 µg desogestrel	28 tablets

*Equivalent to 37.5 µg levonorgestrel.
§Cerazette is a new POP — see p. 67.

Studies are suggestive, but not conclusive, that the failure rate of the POP may be higher with increasing weight, as is well established for progestogen rings and some implants. Pending more data, and given the great medical safety of the method, at the MPC we now usually offer 2 POPs a day to women over 70 kg (irrespective of height), especially if they are young. This is not of course necessary during established breastfeeding or in older women, particularly above age 45.

Mechanism of action and maintenance of effectiveness

The mechanism of action is complex because of variable interactions between the administered progestogen and the endogenous activity of the woman's ovary. Fertile ovulation is prevented in at least 60% of cycles. In the remainder there is reliance mainly on progestogenic interference with mucus penetrability, backed by some anti-nidatory activity at the endometrium. The starting routines are summarized in Table 9.

Table 9
Starting routines for progestogen-only pills.

Condition before start	Start when?	Extra precautions?
Menstruation	Day 1 of period	No
	Day 2 or later	7 days
Postpartum*		
(a) No lactation	Usually day 21	No
(b) Lactation	Day 21 — maybe later if 100% lactation	No
After induced abortion/miscarriage	Same day	No
After COCs	Instant switch	No
Amenorrhoea (e.g. postpartum)	Any time†	7 days

*Bleeding irregularities minimized by starting after 3–6 weeks.
†If prescriber is confident that no blastocyst or sperm is already in upper genital tract. See page 43, final footnote to Table 7.

Interference with contraceptive activity as a result of missed pills, vomiting or drug interaction is believed to start within as little as 3 hours but is corrected adequately, as far as the mucus is concerned, if renewed pill-taking is combined with extra precautions for just 48 hours. However, in the FPA's leaflet 7 days of extra precautions are recommended. This is very cautious but is consistent with the advice for the COCs and may be logical with regard to the anti-ovulatory effect, which occurs in over half of POP users. By analogy with the COC (but there are no POP data) that effect might be expected to take up to a week to be restored.

During full lactation, the efficacy is so much greater that extra precautions need only be advised if a pill is missed for more than 12 hours. Even this is probably over-cautious during the first 6 months postpartum if there is also amenorrhoea. According to the lactational amenorrhoea method (LAM), even without the POP there is only a 1–2% conception risk if — and *only* if — all three criteria continue to apply — namely:

1. **Amenorrhoea, since the lochia ceased**
2. **Full lactation — the baby's nutrition effectively all from its mother**
3. **Baby not yet 6 months old**

So postcoital contraception would very rarely be indicated for missed POPs during full lactation. But because breast-feeding varies in its intensity, it is usual to advise additional precautions during the next 7 tablet-taking days.

In young and highly fertile women it is advisable to recommend switching back to the COC for greater effectiveness as soon as the infant starts to be weaned, ideally no later than the first bleeding episode.

Broad-spectrum antibiotics do not interfere with the effectiveness of POPs. Another contraceptive method would normally be advised during use of enzyme inducers such as *rifampicin* and *griseofulvin*. For long-term treatments with *enzyme inducers*, increasing the dose is an option: usually to two POPs daily, after consideration of other factors such as weight and age.

Advantages and indications

The indications (WHO 1 or sometimes WHO 2) for POP use are as follows:

- Side effects with, or recognized contraindications to, the combined pill, in particular if oestrogen related. As the POP is thought not to affect blood-clotting mechanisms it may be used by women with a definite history of venous thromboembolism (VTE) — and a whole range of disorders predisposing to arterial or venous disease (pp. 33–34). See also p. 66. *Good counselling and record keeping are essential*
- Smokers above 35 years
- Hypertension, whether COC-related or not, controlled on treatment
- Migraine, including focal aura varieties (the woman may continue to suffer migraines but the fear of an EE-promoted thrombotic stroke is eliminated)
- Diabetes, but caution necessary if amenorrhoea develops (see p. 67)
- Lactation, where the combination is extra effective, as good as the COC would be in non-breastfeeders
- Sickle cell disease
- Obesity, but then usually prescribing 2 pills a day (see text)
- At the woman's choice

During lactation, with all POPs the dose to the infant is believed to be harmless, but this aspect must always be discussed. The least amount of administered progestogen gets into the breast milk if a LNG POP is used. The quantity is the equivalent of only one POP in 2 years, considerably less than the progesterone level found in formula feeds.

Contraindications

Absolute contraindications are few:

- Past or current severe arterial diseases, or very high risk thereof
- Any serious adverse effect of COCs not certainly related solely to the oestrogen (e.g. progestogen allergy, liver adenoma)
- Acute porphyria, if history of actual attack (progestogens as well as oestrogens are believed capable of precipitating these)
- Recent trophoblastic disease until hCG is undetectable in blood as well as urine, but earlier use is acceptable in some countries, including the USA (see p. 16)
- Undiagnosed genital tract bleeding
- Actual or possible pregnancy
- Hypersensitivity to any component

To the above can be added four strong **relative** contraindications (all are in the WHO 3 category):

- Acute porphyria, latent, with no previous attack (and caution, forewarning/monitoring); POP also usable in the non-acute porphyrias
- Sex-steroid-dependent cancer, including breast cancer (the agreement of the relevant hospital consultant should be sought)
- Previous treatment for ectopic pregnancy
- Past symptomatic functional ovarian cysts

Although it is now well established that the risk of ectopic pregnancy is actually reduced among POP users, it can be reduced still further by anovulant methods (e.g. the COC, DMPA, Cerazette (p. 67) or Implanon), or by powerfully reducing the chance of fertilization (LNG IUS). These allow better preservation of the precious remaining fallopian tube, especially in nulliparae. The increased frequency of *symptomatic cysts* with POPs may lead to problems in the differential diagnosis from ectopic pregnancy among POP users with abdominal pains. (Persistent cyst/follicles which are commonly detected on routine ultrasonography can usually be disregarded because they cause no symptoms.)

The remaining **relative** contraindications, in which the POP method is generally WHO 2 and may certainly be used with good supervision, are:

- Past venous thromboembolism or severe risk factors for VTE; some would argue that this is in fact WHO 1. See Indications, above
- Risk factors for arterial disease; more than one risk factor can be present, in contrast to COCs
- Current liver disorder even with persistent biochemical change
- Most other chronic severe systemic diseases
- Enzyme inducers (increase the daily dose, see above)

Follow-up and management of side effects

Blood pressure needs to be monitored once a year, after initial checks during 1 year. When raised during administration of COCs it usually reverts to normal on POPs. Indeed, if it does not do so the woman most probably has essential hypertension.

Apart from the complaint of *breast tenderness*, which is usually transient but may be recurrent and can sometimes be overcome by changing from one POP to another, the main side effect is *menstrual irregularity*. With advance warning this is usually well tolerated. It is helpful to chart a bleeding record in early months, because this highlights the type of problem and usually demonstrates improvement. More than half the women will have a cycle between 25 and 35 days. Even when cycles are short, complaints are rare provided that the bleeding is not heavy. A few women experience prolonged or heavy bleeding, and if this is not relieved by changing the POP another method should be selected (perhaps an implant or the IUS).

Except during full lactation, prolonged spells of *amenorrhoea* occur most often in older women. Once pregnancy is excluded, the amenorrhoea must be the result of anovulation and so signifies very high efficacy. The method can be continued unless there is evidence of hypo-oestrogenism (see below).

There are negligible changes to most *metabolic variables*, presumably because of the low dose and the counteracting effect of endogenous oestrogen still produced by the woman's incompletely suppressed ovaries. This is probably true in most POP-users even if they develop *complete amenorrhoea*, but it may not be true in all, raising as with DMPA concerns about *hypo-oestrogenism*, arterial disease or osteoporosis. Pending more data, at the MPC hypo-oestrogenism is assessed regularly at follow-up, and then routinely after about 5 years of amenorrhoea. The assessment is primarily clinical (dry vagina, loss of libido, vasomotor symptoms). But the fuller DMPA protocol (p. 71) with measurements of oestradiol may be used in selected cases.

Establishing ovarian failure at the menopause is less important than with the COC (p. 57), since the POP is a safe enough product to continue using into the late 50s. However, when a non-contraceptive HRT method is desired, if there is amenorrhoea well above age 50 a blood FSH measurement on POP treatment tends to be high (>30 IU/l) if there is ovarian failure, but low if some form of contraception should still be used. Two high values 6 weeks apart, especially if there are vasomotor symptoms, would make the likelihood of a later ovulation very low. Hence first switching to the POP from the COC (see p. 57) can be a reassuring way to manage that often difficult transition out of the reproductive years.

Cerazette

Cerazette is a new and different POP containing 75 µg of desogestrel, a dose which blocks ovulation, as does Implanon — making it like Implanon, by mouth. While irregular bleeding is still a common problem, it has a relatively high incidence of amenorrhoea compared with all previously marketed POPs. Nevertheless, Cerazette generally permits the ovary to supply adequate (follicular phase) oestradiol levels. A most useful feature is that extra contraception need only be advised if a pill is taken 12 hours late. It is expected to be therapeutic for many women with menstrual disorders, especially dysmenorrhoea and menorrhagia, and possibly also functional cysts, ovulation pain and PMS. It will also be a good option if there is a history of ectopic pregnancy.

Injectables

In the UK the only injectable currently licensed by the CSM for long-term use is Depo-Provera (DMPA), and it has been given additional approval as a first-line contraceptive. It has been repeatedly endorsed by the expert committees of prestigious bodies, such as the International Planned Parenthood Federation and WHO. DMPA is even safer than COCs, in spite of the adverse publicity it often receives.

Anxiety about this method was generated by animal research of very doubtful relevance to humans. The latest WHO data imply that DMPA users have a *reduced risk of cancer*, with no overall increased risk of cancers of the breast, ovary or cervix, and a fivefold reduction in the risk of carcinoma of the endometrium (RR 0.2). There is still the possibility of a weak co-factor effect on breast cancer in young women similar to that with COCs (see pp. 10–14). However, this is unproven and the apparent association may be due to surveillance bias in early years of use by the younger women.

Administration, mechanism of action and effectiveness

There are two injectable agents available: Depo-Provera 150 mg every 12 weeks, and Noristerat (norethisterone oenanthate) 200 mg every 8 weeks, both given by deep intramuscular injection in the first 5 days of the menstrual cycle. The injection sites should not be massaged. If *enzyme inducers* are being taken long term, the injection interval is usually shortened to 10 weeks, and to 8 weeks for *rifabutins*.

The effectiveness of DMPA is extremely high among reversible methods (0–1 failure per 100 woman-years), primarily because it functions by causing anovulation, backed by similar effects on the mucus and endometrium to the COC. For overdue injections see p. 106.

The effects, whether wanted (contraceptive) or unwanted, are *not reversible* for the duration of the injection and this fact, unique among current contraceptives, must be explained to prospective users. They must also be warned that after the last dose conception is commonly delayed: a median delay of 9 months, which is of course only 6 months after cessation of the method. Moreover, a comparative study in Thailand showed that almost 95% of previously fertile users had conceived by 28 months after their last injection, which refutes allegations of permanent infertility caused by the drug.

Timing of the first dose
- In *menstruating women* the first injection should normally be given before day 5 of the cycle. If given later than day 2 we advise 7 days' extra precautions. (See also p. 106 for management of 'overdue' injections)
- If a woman is on the *POP or COC*, and pregnancy has been excluded if she is amenorrhoeic (see pp. 43, 62), the injection can be given any time, and with no added precautions
- *Postpartum* (whether or not the woman is breastfeeding), the first injection should *preferably* be 4–6 weeks after the delivery. Postpartum bleeding is thereby minimized — but much earlier use is sometimes clinically justified. Lactation is not inhibited and the dose to the infant is small and believed to be entirely harmless
- *After miscarriage or termination* of pregnancy (first trimester), the injection is normally given within 7 days of the procedure and no extra precautions are required

Advantages and Indications

DMPA has obvious contraceptive benefits (effective, 'forget-table'), but the data imply that it shares most of the non-contraceptive benefits of the COC described on p. 9, including some protection against pelvic infection.

The main indication is the woman's desire for a highly effective method that is independent of intercourse, when other options are contraindicated or disliked. All progestogen-only injectables may be used in spite of a past history of thrombosis (see earlier comments for the POP), and they are ideal for many women who require effective contraception while waiting for major or leg surgery.

Injectables are positively beneficial in endometriosis, in sickle cell anaemia, for women at risk of PID, and in epilepsy, in which it often reduces the frequency of seizures.

Main unwanted effects

The most significant are irregular bleeding, amenorrhoea and weight gain (the latter can be marked in some cases). Preliminary warning minimizes anxiety about these. Menstrual abnormalities remain the greatest obstacle to any large increase in the method's popularity. *Excessive bleeding* may resolve if the next injection is given early (but not less than 4 weeks since the last dose). At the MPC it is often found that giving additional oestrogen is more successful: either as EE 30 µg (as such, or more usually within a pill formulation) or as natural oestrogen (e.g. Premarin 1.25 mg) if there is a past history of thrombosis or migraine with focal aura. Either is given daily for 21 days, after which there is a withdrawal bleed, and courses may be repeated if an acceptable bleeding pattern does not follow.

Amenorrhoea occurs in most long-term users and is usually very acceptable, with the explanation if necessary that 'menstruation has no excretory health benefits'.

There is a concern, however, that *prolonged hypo-oestro-genism* through use of DMPA (particularly if there is oligo-amenorrhoea) might lead by analogy with premature menopause to some added risk of osteoporosis or, more importantly, arterial disease. There is no proof of this — nor that it is not so. The 1998 WHO study of heart disease in current users was somewhat reassuring, but more data are urgently needed.

In the meantime, at the MPC we use the following protocol:

- After 5 years of DMPA use (earlier if there are possibly relevant symptoms such as hot flushes or loss of libido, and in heavy smokers) this issue is raised
- Given the absence of any proof of risk and all the advantages of the method, some women state they will wish to continue uncomplicatedly with DMPA alone, whatever the result of any test; if so, this view of theirs is simply noted
- Other women state after discussion that they wish anyway to make a change to another method, which will of course restore oestrogen levels, either exogenously (e.g. COC) or from their own ovaries
- In the remainder only, the oestradiol level in a blood sample shortly before the next injection is measured
  - If the result is above 100 pmol/l and there are no symptoms, the woman continues on DMPA and the test might be repeated routinely in 3–5 years; if lower, the test is repeated
  - Two levels under 100 pmol/l are taken as grounds for (preferably) a change of method; or more controversially the use of 'add-back' natural oestrogen HRT, by any chosen route and usually continuously. Since it is *unlicensed*, to use DMPA in this way to protect the uterus from the effects of added oestrogen, this must be on a 'named patient' basis (see pp. 114–115)

Contraindications

The **absolute contraindications** are few, as listed earlier for the POP. The **relative contraindications** are also almost identical except that the frequency of ectopic pregnancies and ovarian cysts is reduced, transforming those WHO 3 conditions for the POP into indications (WHO 1). Some studies show a reduction in HDL cholesterol levels, which combined with the hypo-oestrogenism story above means that arterial disease risk is WHO 2 or even 3 according to degree. There is also that built-in lack of immediate reversibility (see p. 69) which will contraindicate the method for some.

Follow-up

Aside from ensuring the injections take place at the correct intervals (and if not, see p. 106), follow-up is primarily advisory and supportive. Excessive bleeding and amenorrhoea are managed as already described. Blood pressure is normally checked initially, but there is absolutely no need for it to be taken before each dose: the studies fail to show any hypertensive effect. An annual check is reasonable as 'well-woman' care.

Contraceptive implants

The implant route remains useful. Applying the lessons from the media and legal saga which led to withdrawal of Norplant, it is clear that good prior counselling is crucial. Explain the likely changes to the bleeding pattern and the possibility of 'hormonal' side effects (see below). This discussion should be backed by a good (e.g. FPA) leaflet and well-documented.

Implants contain a progestogen in a slow-release carrier, made either of dimethylsiloxane (as in Norplant with 6 implants, and the very similar two-rod Norplant II, now called Jadelle) or ethylene vinyl acetate (EVA; Implanon). Inserted into the medial upper arm, after an initial phase of several weeks giving higher blood levels they deliver almost constant low daily levels of the hormone (Figure 13).

Mechanism of action and effectiveness

At the time of writing Implanon was the only marketed implant in the UK. It works primarily by ovulation inhibition, supplemented by the usual mucus and endometrial effects. It is a single 40 mm rod, just 2 mm in diameter, inserted subdermally far more simply than Norplant straight from a dedicated sterile pre-loaded applicator with a cleverly shaped wide-bore needle (Figure 13), by a simple injection/withdrawal technique. The implant contains 68 mg of

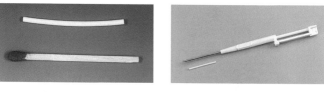

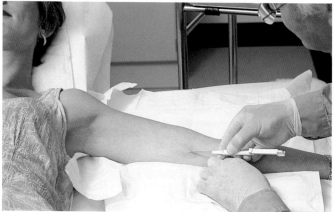

Figure 13
Implanon (by courtesy of Organon Laboratories Ltd).

etonogestrel — the new name for 3-keto-desogestrel. This is dispersed in an EVA matrix and covered by a 0.06 mm rate-limiting EVA membrane.

- The duration of use is for 3 years, with the unique distinction of a zero failure rate in the trials, at the time of writing, though the 95% CI ranges up to 7 in 10 000
- In the international studies serum levels tend to be lower in heavier women, but in my view this should not affect practice — since there have been no failures, whatever the BMI!
- If enzyme inducer drug treatment is necessary, additional contraceptive precautions are recommended.

Though the implant is not difficult to insert or remove, specific training is essential. In a comparative study the mean insertion time was 1.1 minutes (range 0.03–5.00 minutes) and the mean removal time 2.6 minutes (range 0.2–20.00 minutes). This was approximately four times faster for both procedures than for Norplant.

Timing of Implanon insertion
- Day 1–5 of the woman's natural cycle; if later than day 2, at MPC we would recommend additional contraception for 7 days
- Following first-trimester abortion, immediate insertion is best
- Following delivery or second-trimester abortion, insertion on day 21 is recommended, and if later with additional contraception for 7 days. If still amenorrhoeic pregnancy risk should be excluded (p. 43, footnote)
- If breast feeding, the manufacturer urges caution; uncertainty about the probably nil effects of the tiny amount of etonogestrel reaching the breast milk must be discussed (as for the POP)
- Changing from COC or any (other) progestogen-only method, may be inserted on any convenient day; additional barrier method for 7 days advised if the insertion follows a COC-free interval

---

Advantages and indications

The implant would seem especially suitable for women with contraindications to or problems with the COC or other common methods, who want effectiveness without the finality of sterilization. It has much in common with Cerazette (p. 67).

- Above all it provides efficacy and convenience: if the bleeding pattern suits it is a 'forgettable' contraceptive
- Long action with one treatment (3 years), high continuation rates
- Absence of the initial peak dose given orally to the liver
- Blood levels are steady rather than fluctuating (as with the POP) or initially too high (as injectables); this minimizes metabolic changes
- Oestrogen-free, therefore usable if history of VTE (this is WHO 2, in my opinion)
- Median systolic and diastolic blood pressures were unchanged in trials for up to 4 years
- Being an anovulant, special indications include past ectopic pregnancy and all the menstrual disorders which Cerazette (p. 67) may also benefit. A preliminary trial with Cerazette can sometimes be useful
- The implant is rapidly reversible: after removal serum etonogestrel levels were undetectable within 1 week; within 3 weeks 44 out of 47 women were ovulating normally.

Contraindications

Absolute contraindications (WHO 4) are few:

Progestogen-dependent tumours (including active trophoblastic disease, liver adenoma): current breast cancer in WHO 3
Acute porphyria (see p. 65)
Severe hepatic disease with markedly abnormal liver function
Known or suspected pregnancy
Undiagnosed vaginal bleeding
Hypersensitivity to any component

The manufacturer adds 'active venous thromboembolic disorder', but in my view this history (past or present) would be WHO 2. There is no evidence that Implanon would increase the risk.

In my view the **relative contraindications** are as for the POP (p. 65), since, like it but unlike DMPA, Implanon is immediately reversible. They are all WHO 2.

Follow-up and management of side effects

No treatment-specific follow-up is necessary (including no need for BP checks). But there should be an explicit 'open house' policy to discuss possible side effects, without any provider-pressure to persevere if the woman really wants the implant removed.

In the pre-marketing randomized comparative trial of Implanon with Norplant, the *bleeding patterns* were very similar, with one main difference. As expected for an anovulant method, amenorrhoea was significantly more common (20.8 versus 4.4%). The infrequent bleeding and spotting rate was 26.1%. Normal cycling was reported by 35%. But the combined rates for the more annoying 'frequent bleeding and spotting' and 'prolonged bleeding and spotting' totalled 18% with Implanon. The best short-term treatment is cyclical COC therapy, logically with 'Marvelon', after which the bleeding may become acceptable.

'Minor' side effects reported in frequency order were: acne, headache, abdominal pain, breast pain, 'dizziness', mood changes (depression, emotional lability), libido decrease, hair loss. In a comparative study the mean *body weight increase* over 2 years was 2.6% with Implanon and 2.9% with Norplant, but in users of an IUD the weight increase was 2.4%. Though this implies a normal increase over time, by 24 months 35% had put on more than 3 kg. As with DMPA, forewarning about weight is essential: some individuals do put on an unacceptable amount of weight.

Since Implanon suppresses ovulation and does not supply any oestrogen, the same long-term questions as with DMPA arise over *possible hypo-oestrogenism* (p. 71). However, the initial findings on both oestrogen levels and bone density are very reassuring.

Local adverse effects such as infection of the site, migration, difficult removal and scarring are very infrequent. Discomfort at insertion and removal can be minimized by good training.

Intrauterine contraception

Copper-bearing devices

There ought by rights to be a truly dramatic 'come-back' for intrauterine devices (IUDs) in the near future. Women in their thirties have not been requesting them because they were told, in their twenties, to avoid that method. However, a woman in her later reproductive years with, say, two children is the ideal user, especially if she is not yet sure that her family is complete: the devices have not changed but she has. Currently some doctors are complying too readily with requests for male or female sterilization which originate partly out of myths about this alternative. Leaving aside the significant advance represented by the LNG IUS, too few women know that the latest *copper* IUDs are in practice more, not less, effective than the COC.

Advantages of copper IUDs
- Safe: mortality 1:500 000
- Effective: immediately
  postcoitally — unlike the LNG IUS
  highly, with Gyne T 380, cumulative failures at 5 years only 1.4/100 women
- No link with coitus
- No tablets to remember
- Continuation rates high and duration of use can exceed 10 years
- Reversible — even when removed for one of the recognized complications

---

The first choice copper IUD for a parous woman is an available version of the TCu 380/Copper T 380 (Figure 14). This is more than four times as effective (Figure 15) as the Nova T in preventing both intrauterine and (dangerous) ectopic pregnancies. Unlike that largely outdated option, it retains its efficacy with the passage of time (Figure 15). See, however, p. 99.

There is now the Nova T 380, with a greater surface area of copper wire. The manufacturer claims an overall efficacy (Pearl rate) of 0.6/100 woman-years, which still falls short of the TCU 380, though there have been no large comparative studies. The Multiload, even in its 375 thicker wire version, was also significantly less effective than the TCu 380 in the WHO studies, and they found no evidence of the expected better expulsion rate (compare GyneFix, p. 94).

Mechanism of action

In studies, fertilized ova are almost never retrievable from the genital tract of copper IUD users, hence they must operate mainly by preventing fertilization. Their effectiveness when put in postcoitally indicates that they can also

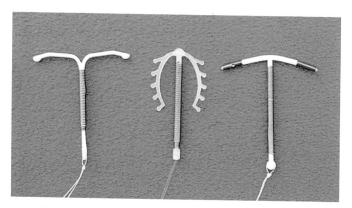

Figure 14
The Nova T, Multiload and Gyne T 380 Slimline version of the TCu 380 IUD. (Reproduced with kind permission of Dr G Cardy). See p. 94 for GyneFix.

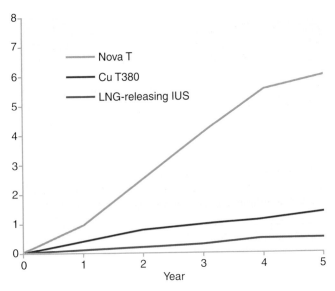

Figure 15
Five-year cumulative gross pregnancy rate per 100 women for 937 women using Nova T; 1821 women using a 20 µg/24 hours levonorgestrel-releasing device; and 1121 women using the Copper-T 380 (recruited in a separate Population Council trial, Sivin et al 1991; rest of data from Andersson et al 1994, European multi-centre trial).

act to block implantation. However, this seems to be primarily a back-up mechanism when devices are *in situ* long term.

As in any given cycle this IUD might be working through the block of implantation, there is a small risk of 'iatrogenic' conception if a device is removed after mid-cycle. Ideally, therefore, women should use another method additionally from 7 days before planned device removal, or removal should be postponed until the next menses. If a device must be removed earlier (e.g. when treating infection) then hormonal postcoital contraception may be indicated.

Influence of age

Copper IUDs, like all contraceptive methods, are more effective in the older woman because of declining fertility. Over the age of 30 there is also a reduction in rates of expulsion and of pelvic inflammatory disease, which is not believed to be the result of the older uterus resisting infection but because the older woman is generally less exposed to risk of infection (through her own lifestyle or that of her only partner).

Adverse effects of copper IUDs

The main medical problems are listed in the Box. This is a remarkably short list as compared with hormonal methods.

Main problems with copper IUDs
- Intrauterine pregnancy — hence miscarriage risks
- Extrauterine pregnancy
- Expulsion — hence the risks of pregnancy/miscarriage
- Perforation — risks of pregnancy
  — risks to bowel/bladder
- Infection
- Pain
- Bleeding — increased amount
  — increased duration

Note: all the first five problems above have the risk of *impairing future fertility*. Moreover they must be excluded as diagnoses before pain and bleeding are ascribed to the method as 'side effects'

In situ conception

If the woman wishes to go on to full term, after a pelvic ultrasound scan the device should normally be removed. This is counterintuitive because one would think it would increase the miscarriage rate. In fact the data for all devices studied show that the miscarriage rate is at least halved by removal of the device in the first trimester. For example, with the Copper T 200 device the normal rate of spontaneous abortion was 55%, dropping to 20% if the device was removed. The woman should of course be warned that an increased risk of miscarriage still remains. Obviously the device should be left for removal at surgery if the woman is going to have a termination of pregnancy. If the threads are already missing when she is seen and other causes are excluded (see below), the pregnancy is at increased risk of second trimester abortion (which could be infected) and antepartum haemorrhage and premature labour.

If the woman goes on to full term it is essential to identify the device in the products of conception; if it is not found, a postpartum X-ray should be arranged in case the device is embedded or has perforated. There have been medicolegal cases when this was not done, leading either to symptoms from an undiagnosed perforation or to unnecessary tests and treatments for 'infertility' when only one IUD was removed for a wanted pregnancy (leaving a much earlier embedded device).

There is no evidence of associated teratogenicity with conception during or immediately after use of copper devices or indeed of cancer developing in the uterus of long-term users.

IUDs with 'lost threads'

The threads are in fact often present, although perhaps short or drawn up into the canal. If not, this symptom of 'lost threads' links together the first, third and fourth bullet points in the Box on p. 81. There are at least six causes of this condition, three with and three without pregnancy (see Box on p. 83). An intra-abdominal IUD is just as useless at stopping pregnancy as one that has been totally expelled. More commonly the woman is already pregnant (and the threads have been drawn up) or the device has altered its position *in situ*. So the slogan is:

> The woman with 'lost threads' is either already pregnant or may be at risk of becoming pregnant

Pregnant	**Not pregnant**
Unrecognized expulsion + pregnancy	Unrecognized expulsion + not yet pregnant
Perforation + pregnancy	Perforation + not yet pregnant
Device *in situ* + pregnancy	Device *in situ* + malpositioned or threads short (in uterus, if not found in cervical canal)

Once pregnancy has been excluded the management is that summarized in Figure 16. First, insert a long-handled Spencer–Wells forceps into the cervical canal and open the jaws carefully under direct vision. The threads were found this way in about 40% of the women referred to the specialized 'lost threads' clinic at the MPC — meaning that they need never have been referred. In most of the remainder the thread was drawn down and the device removed using either the Emmett retriever or the Retrievette. Appropriate analgesia is important: as a routine we give mefenamic acid 500 mg about 30 minutes before the examination but, in addition, local anaesthesia should be offered (see below).

If these manoeuvres fail, referral to the hospital gynaecologist may be necessary. In the study at the MPC only 2.5% of 350 *in situ* intrauterine devices required general anaesthesia for removal, and a similarly low rate should be the norm. Investigations that may be helpful include ultrasound scan and an X-ray (another IUD may usefully be inserted as a uterine marker).

Perforation has a general estimated risk whether for framed or frameless devices of about 1 per 1000 insertions, but the exact rate depends crucially on the skill of the clinician. Perforated devices should now almost always be removed at laparoscopy.

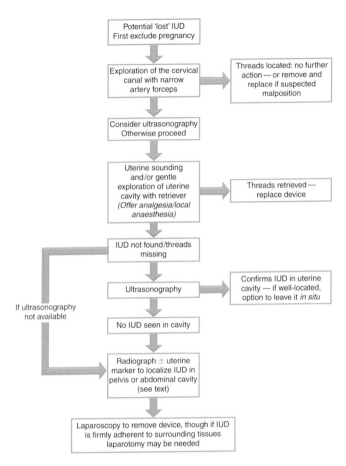

Figure 16
Management of 'lost' IUD threads.

Infection

This is the great fear we all have about intrauterine devices. Just as the pill has been blamed for problems we now know were due to smoking, copper IUDs have been blamed for infections that were really acquired sexually.

Much of the anxiety derived from the Dalkon Shield disaster — but this was a unique device with a polyfilamentous thread, increasing the risk of transfer of potential pathogens from the lower to the upper genital tract. Modern copper devices have a monofilamentous thread. They provide no protection against PID (in contrast to the LNG IUS — see below) and the infections that occur may perhaps be more severe as a result of the foreign body effect, yet they do not themselves cause infection.

The WHO study by Farley et al (1992) reinforces the above view. They reported on a database from WHO RCTs including approximately 23 000 insertions worldwide, and in every country the same pattern emerged (Figure 17). There was an IUD-associated increased risk of infection for 20 days after the insertion. However the weekly infection rate 3 weeks after insertion went back to the same weekly rate as before insertion, i.e. the norm for that particular society. In China there were no infections diagnosed at all in spite of 4301 insertions.

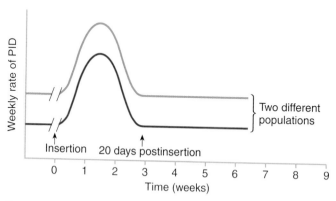

Figure 17

WHO study of 22 908 IUD insertions (4301 in China) in Europe, Africa, Asia and the Americas. PID, pelvic inflammatory disease. Note the weekly rate of PID returns to the preinsertion background rate for the population studied.

These findings are interpreted as follows: the postinsertion infection bulge cannot be the result of bad insertion technique, restricted to doctors outside China. Much more probably, although the doctors in all the centres were searching for truly monogamous couples, they were only successful in this search in China (during the 1980s; China is not unique in this respect today). In the other countries PID-causing organisms (especially *Chlamydia trachomatis*) are presumed to have been present in a proportion of the women. The process of insertion would interfere with natural defensive mechanisms (as confirmed through instrumentation in other contexts, such as therapeutic abortion). This would enable organisms to spread from the lower genital tract, where they had previously resided, into the upper genital tract including the fallopian tubes.

To summarize these WHO findings:

1 The greatest risk is in the first 20 days, possibly caused by pre-existing carriage of sexually transmitted infections.
2 Risk thereafter, as with preinsertion, relates to the background risk of STIs (high in Africa, but so low in mainland China in the late 1980s that it seems to have been virtually absent in the study population).

The slogan is:

> Elective IUD insertions and **reinsertions** should always occur through a 'Chinese cervix' — meaning one established to be pathogen-free

The practical implications are:

- Prospective IUD users should ideally be screened, at least for *Chlamydia trachomatis*, before all IUD insertions or reinsertions
- Exposure history or evidence of a purulent discharge from the cervix indicates more detailed investigation, ideally at a genitourinary medicine clinic
- If *Chlamydia* is detected it should be treated (e.g. doxycycline 100 mg twice daily for 7 days), contact tracing arranged and IUD insertion postponed. In emergency contraception cases (pp. 102–103) screen but treat anyway before the result is available (e.g. with azithromycin 1 g stat)
- The cervix should be cleansed very thoroughly (primarily physically, by swabbing) before the device is inserted, with minimum trauma following the manufacturer's instructions
- In addition to the routine 6-week follow-up visit, a first postinsertion visit should logically be arranged after 7 days, designed to identify any women with postinsertion infection (during the 'hump' of Figure 17). As a minimum, the woman should be given clear details of the relevant symptoms of PID, and instructed as a routine to telephone the practice nurse about a week postinsertion

The sexual history, particularly of a new partner in the previous 6 months, is of relevance, although never sufficient. In a study at the MPC during the mid 1980s the background rate of *Chlamydia* carriage was 2.4% in the general clinic population, but higher, 8.2%, in the pre-IUD group who had first been sensitively questioned about their exposure risk. Thus in the UK today it is surely suboptimal to fit IUDs or IUSs without microbiological screening. The added expenses of screening and the antibiotics are readily justified in the context of the Gyne T 380: an annual cost of about £1 per year over 10–13 years makes it such a bargain. 'Blind' prescription of an appropriate antibiotic is necessary in emergency cases, but the screening should still be done. Otherwise contact tracing is impossible and reinfection (possibly worsened by the IUD foreign body effect) will simply occur later.

Actinomyces-like organisms

These organisms (ALOs) are frequently reported in cervical smears, more commonly with increasing duration of use of the device. If there are relevant symptoms (excessive discharge, pain, dyspareunia, tenderness) or signs then the device should be removed and sent for culture, with a low threshold for hospital referral. Treatment will have to be vigorous, usually prolonged, if pelvic actinomycosis is actually confirmed — it is a potentially life-threatening condition, although very rare.

More usually the finding occurs in asymptomatic women. In a study reported from the MPC in 1984 three groups of women were followed up: one group was simply monitored (and the ALO finding commonly persisted), and in two groups the device was removed with or without immediate reinsertion of another copper IUD. In both these second two groups follow-up smears were free of ALOs. As a result, simple removal with reinsertion has become the usual practice at the MPC, without antibiotic treatment. A cervical smear is repeated after 6 months, then at normal intervals. Meticulous 6-monthly follow-up, including a check for symptoms and bimanual examination of asymptomatic women, is the other management option (especially perhaps for the LNG IUS, pp. 95–99), so long as they are advised (including written reference material) about the relevant symptoms which should make them seek urgent medical advice. While the original IUD/IUS remains *in situ*, cervical smears are bound to continue showing the ALOs; they are repeated at normal screening intervals.

Ectopic pregnancy
Is this problem caused by copper IUDs? This also appears to be a myth. The main cause is previous tubal infection with one or both tubes being damaged. The non-causative association with IUDs comes about because they tend to be even more effective at preventing pregnancy in the uterus than in the tube. Therefore the ratio of extra- to intrauterine pregnancies is higher than expected. Ectopic pregnancies are actually reduced in number because very few sperm get through the copper-containing uterine fluids to reach an

egg, so very few implantations can occur, in any damaged tube. However, there are even fewer implantations in the uterus. Thus in the ratio of ectopic to intrauterine pregnancies, the denominator is even lower than the numerator, allowing the ratio to increase — even though both types of pregnancy are actually reduced in frequency. The estimated rate of ectopic pregnancy for sexually active Swedish women seeking pregnancy is (1.2–1.6/100 woman-years). The risk in users of the Gyne T 380 and its clones is estimated as 0.02/100 woman-years, which is at least 60 times lower. But the ectopic rate for the Nova T (old version) is not so good, about 0.25/100 woman-years, another reason to prefer the Gyne T 380.

Clinically, caution about ectopic pregnancy is still necessary:

> Any IUD user with pain and a late period or irregular bleeding has an ectopic pregnancy until proved otherwise. A past history is a relative contraindication (WHO 3) to the method (see below), particularly in nulliparae

Pain and bleeding

As already stressed:

> Pain and bleeding in IUD users signify a dangerous condition until proved otherwise

As well as excluding conditions such as infection and an ectopic pregnancy or miscarriage, malposition of any framed device (contrast GyneFix, see below) can cause pain through uterine spasms.

Copper devices do increase the duration of bleeding by a mean of 1–2 days, and they also increase the measured volume of bleeding by about a third. In a population of copper IUD users haemogloblin levels tend to fall, and those with losses above 80 ml/cycle are prone to frank anaemia. Bleeding problems usually settle with time. If they do not it may be necessary to change the method of contraception, perhaps to the LNG IUS method (see below). Drug treatments may reduce the loss but are not very satisfactory long term. The most successful therapies are mefenamic acid 500 mg 8-hourly and tranexamic acid 1–1.5 g 8-hourly.

Which device?
The TCu 380 and GyneFix (p. 94) appear to be the most effective copper IUDs available, at least twice as effective in the first year of use, and four or five times as effective cumulatively over 5 years, as the Nova T. Indeed, the Copper T 380 first year failure rate was brilliant, about 0.4/100 woman-years. No pregnancies at all were detected beyond 5 years' use — in marked contrast to the Nova T (see Figure 15), though it is likely that the Nova T 380, loaded with additional copper, will perform better. GyneFix is for women expected to benefit from its low risk of expulsion, malposition and frame-related pain. We have no experience at MPC with the new Flexi-T 300. It appears useful for small uteri, and in a 1995 RCT was as effective as TCu 380. For Multiload IUDs see pp. 79, 99.

Duration of use
Studies show reduced rates of discontinuation with increasing duration of use, whether for expulsion, infection or bleeding and pain. Coupled with the fact that most IUD complications are insertion-related, it is good news that the Cu T 380 is now fully approved for 10 years of use in the UK and 13 years in the USA. As it is a similarly *banded* IUD, I am confident the GyneFix will eventually be usable for at least as long. Nova T devices should be removed on efficacy grounds after 3 years (or maximum 5 years) in all women under 40.

The agreed policy **above age 40**, since a 1990 statement in *The Lancet* by the FPA and the predecessor body of the Faculty of Family Planning and Reproductive Health Care, is:

Any copper device which has been fitted above the age of 40 may be that woman's last device and never needs to be changed. (But it may not be so licensed, see pp. 114–115)

Which user?

Main established contraindications to copper IUDs (contrast p. 98)
Absolute (WHO 4): but perhaps temporary

1. Suspected pregnancy
2. Unexplained uterine bleeding
3. Current or very recent active pelvic infection or significant pelvic tenderness, or purulent cervical discharge
4. Recent proven STI, unless fully investigated, treated and contacts traced (to provide a 'Chinese cervix', see p. 86)
5. Significant immunosuppression (not standard oral corticosteroid therapy)
6. Malignant trophoblastic disease with uterine wall involvement on ultrasound scan

Absolute (WHO 4) and permanent

7. Distorted uterine cavity or cavity < 5.5 cm (NB not necessarily a problem with GyneFix (WHO 2))
8. Wilson's disease (copper devices only)
9. Known true allergy to a constituent
10. Heart valve prosthesis, or past attack of bacterial endocarditis

Relative contraindications (WHO 2 unless otherwise stated)
LNG IUS often preferred choice when they apply
A copper IUD is usable with caution:

1. Structural heart disease (bacterial endocarditis risk without history); full antibiotic cover should be given to cover the insertion
2. Hip replacement or other non-heart-valve prosthesis which could be prejudiced by blood-borne infection (antibiotic cover)
3. Past history of ectopic pregnancy or other history suggesting high ectopic risk in a multipara (WHO 3), (Cu T 380, GyneFix or LNG IUS are preferred IUDs; but even better to use an anovulant contraceptive). In young nulliparae some still consider this an absolute contraindication
4. Past history of definite PID
5. Lifestyle risking STIs
6. Known HIV infection (WHO 3, LNG IUS preferred)
7. Questionable fertility for any reason
8. Nulliparity/young age (GyneFix and LNG IUS have been used electively and very successfully in selected research populations of nulliparae)
9. Severely scarred or mildly distorted uterus (e.g. after myomectomy)

Counselling (by doctor or nurse)

After considering the contraindications, there should be an unhurried discussion with the woman of the main points above, particularly regarding her infection risk, the failure rate and the importance of reporting pain as a symptom. The woman should always be given a user-friendly back-up leaflet, and assured that in the event of relevant symptoms she will receive prompt advice and, as indicated, a pelvic examination. *Timing* of insertions must avoid an implanted pregnancy (p. 102) but otherwise can be at any time and usually 6 weeks postpartum (beware increased risk of perforation).

Insertion of devices

A pocketbook such as this is not the right medium for teaching insertion techniques. The Faculty training leading to the Letter of Competence in Intrauterine Contraception Techniques is strongly recommended. This is a one-to-one apprenticeship, supplemented by videos and practice with an appropriate pelvic model, following the illustrations in each packet. Training should include more attention than in the past to the issue of analgesia; at the MPC women routinely receive mefenamic acid 500 mg while in the waiting room. Local anaesthesia by intracervical injection should be taught, and offered as a choice. It should almost always be used if the cervix has to be dilated or the uterine cavity explored. Lignocaine jelly 2% (Instillagel) inserted by quill is under evaluation but so far seems to be somewhat less effective (though more comfortable to insert) than a cervical block — as well as raising questions about upward transfer of organisms from the cervix.

Once learned, the skills — including management of 'lost threads' — must be maintained by regular practice. Note that:

> Insertion can be a factor in the causation of almost every category of IUD problems. Another reason to prefer long-lived devices!

Copper IUD summary

1	Last 9 days of the cycle	Time of one of the main actions (which might be operative)
2	Main counselling point	Fertility (risk and importance thereof)
3	Pregnancy, expulsion and infection	All less common with increasing age
4	Most IUD problems	Insertion related
5	Continuing *in situ* pregnancy	Gently remove IUD in first trimester
6	Pain + irregular bleeding	Ectopic pregnancy or other serious cause?
7	'Lost threads'	Pregnant or at risk until proved otherwise
8	Duration of use	Long-term use is best* — 'leave well alone', especially to avoid the risks of each new insertion

*Except: after 3–5 years if a Nova T was fitted under age 40, or with any IUD if ALOs detected — see above.

GyneFix

This unique frameless device (Figure 18) features a knot, which is embedded by its special inserter system in the fundal myometrium. Below the knot, its polypropylene thread bears six copper bands and locates them within the uterine cavity. It appears to retain the efficacy and other advantages of the Cu T 380, but once properly implanted has a much lower expulsion rate (0.4/100 woman-years in the first year of use) and no removals for pain of mechanical origin. Malpositioning is also less likely than with framed IUDs. Special training for the implantation is essential, even by doctors accustomed to inserting the existing devices. A new inserter mechanism to reduce perforation risk is under evaluation.

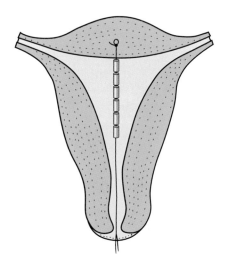

Figure 18
The GyneFix intrauterine copper implant. A hybrid, with this superb new implantation technique but releasing LNG or another potent progestogen, is a highly desirable future development.

The levonorgestrel-releasing intrauterine system (LNG IUS)

This Nova T-shaped device is shown in Figure 19. Note that:

- It releases 20 µg/24 hours of LNG from its polydimethylsiloxane reservoir through a rate-limiting membrane, over at least 5 years
- Its main contraceptive effects are local, through changes to the cervical mucus and uterotubal fluid which impair sperm migration, backed by endometrial changes impeding implantation
- The systemic blood levels of LNG are under half of the mean levels in users of the POP, and so ovarian function is altered less
- Most women continue to ovulate and in the remainder sufficient oestrogen is produced from the ovary even if they become amenorrhoeic as many do, primarily through a local end-organ effect
- Return of fertility is rapid and appears to be complete
- It is highly convenient and has few adverse side effects
- It is in short a contraceptive in which the default state is one of contraception, unlike pills and condoms where the default state is the reverse — conception

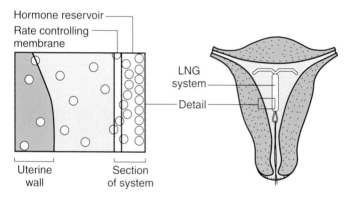

Figure 19
The LNG-releasing IUS (Mirena).

The above advantages are of course shared with the Gyne T 380 which is the current 'gold standard' for copper IUDs. However, this is where the similarity ends. It fundamentally 'rewrites the textbooks' about IUDs, really only sharing the intrauterine location and deserving a separate category (hence 'IUS'). The user of this method can expect:

a dramatic reduction in amount and, after the first few months (discussed below), duration of blood loss

Dysmenorrhoea and (for unexplained reasons) the premenstrual syndrome (PMS) are frequently improved. The LNG IUS is the contraceptive method of choice for most women with heavy menses or who are prone to iron-deficiency anaemia. It should be the first-line long-term primary care treatment for excessively heavy menses — for which it is fully licensed in all circumstances except where contraception will never be required (i.e. only when the woman has herself been sterilized).

By providing progestogenic protection of the uterus during oestrogen replacement by any chosen route it uniquely, before final ovarian failure, offers 'forgettable, contraceptive, no-period and no PMS-type HRT'. Although not yet licensed for the latter in the UK it may be used on a 'named patient' basis (pp. 114–115), but not left *in situ* above 5 years.

What about infection/ectopics/risk to future fertility?

Although existing IUDs do not themselves cause PID, they fail to prevent it and they tend to worsen the attacks that occur (see above). The LNG IUS may actually reduce the frequency of clinical PID, particularly in the youngest age groups who are most at risk. The risk is certainly not eliminated, but the data available make it possible to offer the LNG IUS to some young women requesting a default state contraceptive who would not be good candidates for conventional copper IUDs. 'ALOs' may be reported, and the finding should be managed as described on p. 88.

The Progestasert and an experimental WHO device that released only 2 µg/day of levonorgestrel were both associated with an *increased* risk of extrauterine pregnancies. The data on file and published for this device show (as for the banded copper IUDs) a definite *reduction* in that risk, which can be attributed to its greater efficacy by mechanisms that reduce the risk of pregnancy in any site, whether uterine or extrauterine.

Main adverse effects of the LNG IUS

As with any intrauterine device expulsion can occur and there is the usual small risk of *perforation*, minimized by its 'withdrawal' as opposed to 'plunger' technique of insertion. An improved insertion system is expected soon.

A more important problem is the high incidence in the first postinsertion months of *uterine bleeding* which, although small in quantity, may be very frequent or continuous and can cause considerable inconvenience. Later in the use of the method amenorrhoea is commonly reported. For both these effects, particularly the first, forewarned is forearmed — implying the need for good counselling. In my experience, women can accept the early weeks of frequent light bleeding as a worthwhile price to pay for all the other advantages of the method, if they are well informed in advance of LNG IUS fitting, and coached and encouraged as appropriate while it is occurring. The amenorrhoea can be explained and interpreted to a woman as an advantage — not an adverse side effect but a positive benefit of the method.

Women should also be forewarned that, although this method is mainly local in its action, it is not exclusively so. Therefore there is a small incidence of 'hormonal' side effects such as bloatedness, acne and depression. These do usually improve, often within 2 months, in parallel with the known decline in the higher initial LNG blood levels. Some clinicians find that early removals for this particular reason can be minimized by each woman having a short preliminary trial with a LNG-containing POP.

Functional ovarian cysts are also more common, although they are usually asymptomatic. If pain results they should be investigated/monitored and will usually resolve spontaneously.

Contraindications to the LNG IUS

There are very few absolute contraindications:

> - Hypersensitivity to levonorgestrel
> - Suspected pregnancy
> - Unexplained uterine bleeding
> - Current active pelvic infection or pelvic tenderness, or purulent cervical discharge
> - Recent proven STI, unless fully investigated and treated
> - Severely distorted uterine cavity, or measuring <5.5 cm. The IUS may be usable subsequent to hysteroscopic removal of a submucous fibroid. The implantable variant mentioned on p. 94 would be so valuable here!
> - Severe immunodeficiency (not steroid therapy)
> - Past attack of bacterial endocarditis or any prosthetic heart valve
> - Any current active trophoblastic disease with raised hCG
> - Current active hepatocellular disease or liver tumour
> - Current active arterial disease
>
> Note: the last three bullets relate to LNG-hormonal actions and are WHO 3 at most in my view.
>
> **In addition**:
> - The LNG IUS should not be used as a postcoital intrauterine contraceptive (a failure has been reported, and it may not act quite rapidly enough). Until more data are available copper IUDs (e.g. GyneFix) should normally be used for that indication

Almost all the relative contraindications listed above (pp. 91–91) for copper IUDs apply to the LNG IUS but are less strong (certainly no more than WHO 2), and bleeding and pain are of course positive indications (WHO 1).

Insertion of the LNG IUS

The technique is almost identical to that for the Nova T. However, the insertion tube is wider (4.8 mm), meaning that a set of Hegar size 3–6 dilators should always be available and the skills for effective local anaesthesia may quite frequently be required. This again highlights the importance of good training (a video is available from the manufacturer), and of maintaining experience.

Conclusions

This method fulfils many of the standard criteria for an ideal contraceptive (Box). It approaches 100% reversibility, effectiveness and even, after some delay, convenience. This is because, after the initial months of frequent uterine bleedings and spotting, the usual outcomes of either intermittent light menses or amenorrhoea are very acceptable to most women. Adverse side effects are few and in general they are in the nuisance category rather than hazardous. Evidence continues to accumulate of the non-contraceptive benefits previously described, and others are emerging.

Since the advent of the LNG IUS my own lecture entitled 'Contraception for older women and those with intercurrent diseases' has been considerably simplified.

However, this method does require initial and some ongoing medical interventions and also fails against the fifth criterion in the Box below. There is no known protection against sexually transmitted viruses (and no *complete* protection against other STIs). So the 'Double-Dutch' approach (see p. 4) remains relevant.

The ideal contraceptive
- 100% reversible
- 100% effective (with the default state as contraception)
- 100% convenient (and non-coitally related)
- 100% free of adverse side effects (neither risk nor nuisance)
- 100% protective against sexually transmitted infections
- Has other non-contraceptive benefits
- Maintenance free (needing no ongoing medical intervention)

Postscript The excellent Gyne T 380 IUD was withdrawn by its manufacturer (on commercial grounds), and efforts to replace it with a near-identical TCu 380 'clone' may take some while. Acceptable alternative framed IUDs for the interim are: the Multiload 375 (not the 250 or Short, and used for parous women only); the Nova T 380 (not the Nova T, p. 79) and the Flexi-T 300. See pp. 79, 89, 90. The indications for GyneFix and Mirena are unchanged.

The use of large doses of oestrogen is outmoded because of severe nausea and vomiting. Apart from mifepristone, still unavailable for this use, three methods have now been shown to be effective: the insertion of a copper IUD, the combined oral emergency contraceptive (COEC) marketed as Schering PC4 and, most recently, the LNG-containing progestogen-only emergency contraceptive (POEC) (Table 10). Marketed as Levonelle 2, POEC has effectively made COEC of largely historical interest only.

An important new finding for both hormone methods is that every 12 hours' delay in treatment increases the failure rate by 50%. Awkwardly for providers, this takes us back to the concept of the 'morning after pill', indicating somewhat of an 'emergency'. 'Emergency pill' remains a better lay term, since it leaves open the fact that useful benefit can be obtained up to at least 72 hours (Table 11). The POEC is already available over the counter in some countries (e.g. Norlevoin in France) and in the UK discussions are in progress about the appropriate safeguards.

POEC — one hormone is best!

In the 1998 RCT by WHO, comparing around 1000 women given this method (POEC) and the same number given COEC after a single exposure, the main findings were as in

Table 10
Choice of methods for postcoital contraception.

	POEC (Levonelle 2) Levonorgestrel 0.75 mg ×2 12 hours apart	**COEC (Schering PC4)** 0.25 mg LNG +50 µg EE ×2 tablets ×2 doses 12 hours apart	**Copper IUD** Immediate insertion
Normal timing after intercourse	Up to 72 hours	Up to 72 hours	Up to 5 days after earliest calculated day of ovulation (see page 102)
Efficacy (overall) (WHO study)	99%	97%	About 99.9%
Side effects	Nausea 23% Vomiting 6%	Nausea 51% Vomiting 19%	Pain, bleeding, risk of infection
Contraindications	• Pregnancy • Proven severe acute allergy to a constituent • Active acute porphyria • Active severe liver disease	• Pregnancy • Proven severe acute allergy to a constituent • Active acute porphyria • Active severe liver disease • Current focal migraine • Current sickle cell crisis	• Pregnancy • As for copper IUDs generally

Reference: WHO, *Lancet* 1998; 352:428–33. Numbers rounded to nearest integer.
LNG = levonorgestrel; EE = ethinyloestradiol. See also p. 16.

Table 11
Relative efficacies in each 24-hour period.

Coitus to treatment interval	**POEC (Levonelle 2)**		**COEC (Schering PC4)**	
	Failure rate among all-comers %	% of expected pregnancies prevented	Failure rate among all-comers %	% of expected pregnancies prevented
<24 hours	0.4	95	2	77
25–48 hours	1.2	85	4.1	36
49–72 hours	2.7	58	4.7	31

Note: On the basis of previous research into conception probabilities, 92 out of each 100 presenting in the study would not have conceived after the single exposure if untreated. 'Expected pregnancies' therefore use the remaining 8% as the denominator.

Tables 10 and 11. The main advantages of POEC are reduced rates of nausea and vomiting; it is also more effective (99.6% when treatment began within 24 hours, compared with 98% for COEC — in the circumstances of the WHO trial); and in ordinary practice there are virtually no contraindications to it apart from existing pregnancy.

Contraindications
Absolute contraindications to the hormone methods are few and listed in Table 10. There is no upper age limit to any of the methods if sufficient risk of conception is present.

If the woman is taking an *enzyme-inducer drug* (including St John's Wort), the doses with either of the hormonal methods should be increased by 50% (i.e. a third tablet of POEC). No increase in dose is recommended when *antibiotics* are in use, aside of course from *rifampicin/rifabutin* and *griseofulvin* because they induce liver enzymes.

Copper IUD

Insertion *in good faith* of a copper IUD — not the LNG IUS (see p. 98) — before implantation, which is up to 5 days after the (earliest) calculated ovulation day, is extremely effective and prevents conception in almost 100% of women — even in cases of multiple exposure. The judge's summing up in a 1991 Court Case (Regina vs Dhingra) gives legal support to this policy:

> 'I further hold . . . that a pregnancy cannot come into existence until the fertilized ovum has become implanted in the womb, and that that stage is not reached until, at the earliest, the 20th day of a normal 28 day cycle . . .'

Contraindications
There are recognized contraindications and risks of pain, bleeding or infection, as with any intrauterine method, so this option is not often advised for the nulliparous woman. However, in selected cases after cervical swabs (for *Chlamydia trachomatis* at least) and prophylactic antibiotic

cover (p. 87), and contact tracing if the bacteriology is positive, it may be appropriate.

Indications for emergency contraception by copper IUD

- When maximum efficacy is the woman's priority
- When exposure occurred more than 72 hours earlier, or in cases of multiple exposure: insertion may be up to 5 days after ovulation
- In many parous women, to be retained as their long-term method (although it may be right in young women to remove it once they are established on a new method such as the COC or injectable)
- Presence of absolute contraindications to either hormonal method (a very rare indication since POEC)
- After vomiting of either dose within 2 hours, in a case with particularly high pregnancy risk

Summary: counselling and management

First, evaluate the possibility of sexual assault or rape. Then:

1   Careful assessment of menstrual/coital history, and hence of the appropriateness of treatment, is essential. Other exposures to risk earlier than the one presented with need particular consideration.
2   The mode of action sometimes (not always) being post-fertilization may pose an absolute contraindication to some individuals. Most modern ethicists (and this author) consider that blocking of implantation is contraception, not abortion.
3   Medical risks should be discussed, especially:
    – the failure rate (see Table 11), but remind the woman that these figures relate to a single exposure. The failure rate is very close to nil for the IUD method.
    – teratogenicity: this is believed to be negligible — although there is no proof — because before implantation the hormones will not reach the blastocyst in sufficient concentration to cause any adverse effect. Follow-up of women who have kept their pregnancies

has so far not shown any increased risk of major abnormalities above the background 2% rate.

– ectopic pregnancy: if this occurs it is the result of a pre-existing damaged tube and would almost certainly have happened anyway, with or without this (pre-implantation) treatment. However, a past history of ectopic pregnancy or pelvic infection remains a reason for caution and forewarning with any of the methods.

4   Even if the POEC method is used, advice should be given regarding nausea and vomiting (the latter occurs in 6% of cases). If an anti-emetic is requested, the best seems to be domperidone (Motilium), 10 mg with each dose. If either contraceptive dose is vomited within 2 hours, the woman may be given further tablets or, in a particularly high-risk case, a copper IUD should be inserted.

5   Contraception both in the current cycle (in case the POEC method merely postpones ovulation) and long term should be discussed. The IUD option covers both aspects. If the COC is chosen it should be started as soon as the woman is convinced her next period is normal, usually on the first or second day, without the need for additional contraception thereafter.

The above makes clear the importance of a good rapport to obtain an accurate coital and menstrual history and to promote effective arrangements for follow-up.

Vaginal examination is rarely necessary and there are very good reasons to omit it, for example, in an anxious teenager. It should be done if indicated in the individual case on clinical grounds:

- At the first visit clinical grounds might be to exclude overt infection or concealed clinical pregnancy and to establish a baseline size and shape for the uterus
- At follow-up, examination is mainly indicated if there is clinical uncertainty because the next period is delayed, or in the presence of any pain

---

Special indications

These apply to coital exposure when the following have occurred:

1 **Omission of 2 or more COC tablets** after the pill-free interval (PFI, see p. 50), or of *any combination of pills from the first 7 in the packet which in the prescriber's judgement amounts to the same thing as lengthening the PFI to 9 or more days.* After the emergency regimen the woman may return immediately to the COC, subject to a 100% undertaking to return for follow-up 4 weeks later — and also to use added precautions for the next 7 days. Mid-packet pill omissions after 7 tablets have been taken never indicate emergency treatment unless at least 4 have been missed. Towards the end of a packet, omission of the next PFI will suffice.

2 **Delay in taking a POP tablet for more than 3 hours**, implying loss of mucus effect, followed by exposure during the 48 hours before contraception is expected to be restored. Again the POP is restarted immediately after the emergency regimen, 7 days' added precautions are advised, and follow-up agreed. If the POP user is fully breastfeeding (p. 63) or the POP in use is Cerazette (p. 67), these actions would only be contemplated if the POP is taken more than 12 hours late.

3 **Removal or expulsion of an IUD** before the time of implantation, if another IUD cannot be inserted for some reason.

4 **Further exposure in the same cycle**, e.g. due to failure of barrier contraception after an emergency hormonal method has been given. Additional courses of POEC, for example, are acceptable (if all are taken before any possible implantation). But this additional use is of course outside the terms of the licence (see pp. 114–115).

5 **Use later than 72 hours after exposure.** Although COEC and POEC have so far been tested only up to 72 hours after the earliest act of unprotected intercourse,

they may also be given later — though with uncertainty about the (diminishing) chance of success, as is clear from Table 11. Neither method should be used if calculations suggest that any earlier act could have led to the presence by now of an early implanted pregnancy.

6 **Overdue injections of DMPA with continuing sexual intercourse**. At the MPC we simply give the next dose from day 85 to 91 (i.e. the thirteenth week), plus condoms to be used during the next 7 days. Later, in addition, we exclude an implanted pregnancy (so far as possible, by the coital history and a sensitive pregnancy test) and offer POEC or a copper IUD. After day 98 (fourteen weeks), the next injection is best postponed until there has been a total of 14 days of safe contraception or abstinence since the last exposure and a sensitive (25 mIU/l) pregnancy test is negative (see p. 43).

In all circumstances of use of emergency contraception, always counsel the women regarding possible failure and provide no guarantee that any fetus will be normal.

Research continues and alternatives such as mifepristone may supersede the current methods in due course.

Other methods

Barrier methods

Barrier methods are again in fashion. In spite of their well-known disadvantages they all (notably condoms) provide useful protection against sexually transmitted infections. *All users of this type of method should be informed about emergency contraception, in case of lack of use or failure in use.* Vegetable and oil-based lubricants, and the bases for many prescribable vaginal products, can seriously damage and lead to rupture of rubber: baby oil destroys up to 95% of a condom's strength within 15 minutes. Beware *ad hoc* use of substances from the kitchen or bathroom cupboard! Water-based products such as KY jelly, and also glycerine and silicone lubricants, are not suspect. The Durex Information Service has produced a useful leaflet listing common vaginal preparations which should be regarded as unsafe to use with rubber condoms and diaphragms, and there may be others:

Preparations unsafe to use with rubber condoms or diaphragms

Arachis oil enema	Nizoral
Baby oil	Nystan cream (pessaries OK)
Cyclogest	Ortho Dienoestrol
Dalacin cream	Ortho-Gynest (Ovestin OK)
Ecostatin	Petroleum jelly
Fungilin	Premarin cream
Gyno-Daktarin	Sultrin
Gyno-Pevaryl (Pevaryl OK)	Vaseline
Monistat	Witepsol-based preparations

Sheaths or condoms

Condoms are the only proven barrier to transmission of HIV, yet at the time of writing it still remains impossible in the UK for most couples to obtain this life-saver free of charge from their GP. Condoms are second in usage to the pill under the age of 30 and to sterilization above that age. One GP has reported a failure rate as low as 0.4/100 woman-years, but 2–15 is more representative. Failure, often unrecognized at the time, can almost always be attributed to incorrect use, mainly through escape of a small amount of semen either before or after intercourse. Conceptions, particularly among the young or those who have become a bit casual after years of using a simple method such as the COC, can sometimes be 'iatrogenic', because of lack of explanation by nurse or doctor of the basics.

Some are entirely satisfied with the condom, whereas others use it as a temporary or back-up method; for many who have become accustomed to alternatives not related to intercourse it is completely unacceptable. Some older men, or those with sexual anxiety, complain that its use may result in loss of erection; they should perhaps encourage their female partners to use the female condom (see below).

True rubber allergy can also occur, rarely, but is often solved by use of plastic condoms (e.g. Avanti) or non-spermicidal lubricant. Modern rubber condoms have reduced allergenic residues from the manufacturing process. For women who dislike the smell or messiness of semen, the condom solves their problem.

Hopefully the new Ez-On condom recently marketed in The Netherlands will soon be available in the UK. This is a loose-fitting lubricated plastic condom: the 'looks funny, feels good' condom. By simulating the vagina it is designed to overcome the undeniable interference with penile sensation that occurs during the penetration phase of intercourse.

Femidom

Femidom (Figure 20) is a female condom comprising a polyurethane sac with an outer rim at the introitus and a loose inner ring, whose retaining action is similar to that of the rim of the diaphragm. It thus forms a well-lubricated secondary vagina. Available over the counter, along with a well-illustrated leaflet, it is considerably less likely than most male condoms to rupture in use. It is also completely resistant to damage by any chemicals with which it might come into contact. Using it, the penetrative phase of intercourse can start before the man's erection is complete. However, couples should be forewarned of the possibility that the penis may become wrongly positioned between the Femidom sac and the vaginal wall.

Reports about its acceptability are mixed, and a sense of humour certainly helps. There is clear evidence, however, of a group of women (with their partners) who use it regularly; sometimes alternating with the male equivalent ('his

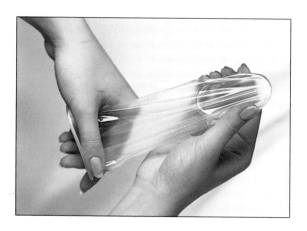

Figure 20
The female condom (Femidom). (Reproduced with kind permission of Chartex International plc.)

night' then 'her night'). As the first female-controlled method with high potential for preventing HIV transmission it must be welcomed.

The cap or diaphragm

Once initiated, many couples express surprise at the simplicity of the diaphragm method, although it is often acceptable only when sexual activity takes on a relatively regular pattern. It may be inserted well ahead of coitus, and so used without spoiling spontaneity. There is very little reduction in sexual sensitivity, as the clitoris and introitus are not affected and cervical pressure is still possible. Spermicide is recommended because no mechanical barrier is complete, although we still lack definitive research on this point. The jelly vehicles (gels) may provide useful lubrication for older women, for those in the postnatal period and for others slow to lubricate as a result of sexual arousal.

The acceptability of the diaphragm depends on the manner and context in which it is offered. Its first-year failure rate, now estimated as 4–8 per 100 careful and consistent users, rising to 10–18 per 100 'typical users' who are less compliant, makes it very unsuitable for most young women who would not accept pregnancy. However, it suits others who are 'spacers' of their family. And it is capable of excellent protection above age 35 (see Table 1), provided it is as well taught and correctly and consistently used as in the Oxford/FPA study.

As for the IUD, for those who wish to offer this choice there is no substitute for one-to-one training in the process of fitting the diaphragm and teaching its correct use, backed by an appropriate leaflet. The woman must learn the vital regular secondary check that she has covered her cervix.

When there is great difficulty in inserting anything into the vagina, be it tampon, pessaries or a cap, obviously the method is not suitable. This problem may be connected with a psychosexual difficulty which may first present during the teaching of the method, but simple lack of anatomical knowledge is often involved. Rejection of a vaginal barrier on account of 'messiness' may also be the result of such a problem. The offer of a less wet-feeling alternative for the spermicide may help, especially Delfen foam.

Follow-up
If either partner complains that they can feel the barrier during coitus the fitting must be urgently checked. It could be too large or too small, or the retropubic ledge may be insufficient to prevent the front slipping down the anterior vagina, or, most seriously, the diaphragm may be being placed regularly in the anterior fornix. The arcing spring diaphragm is then particularly useful.

Chronic cystitis may be exacerbated by pressure from the anterior rim, and the condition often improves with a vault or cervical cap. Diaphragms should be checked annually, postpartum and if there is a 4 kg gain or loss in weight.

Female barriers can be used happily and very successfully by many couples, but high motivation is essential. Once again, a good sense of humour helps.

Spermicides

Although invaluable as adjuncts to caps and condoms, by themselves creams, jellies, pessaries and foams are usually not acceptably reliable (although good pregnancy rates have been obtained in some women, especially during the climacteric).

Delfen foam shares with the contraceptive sponge (at the time of writing, due to be re-launched in the UK) the advantages of being sexually very convenient and unobtrusive in use. Either method can be used by women whose natural fertility is reduced, particularly with increasing age (see Table 1).

Many substances are well absorbed from the vagina, but there is no proof of systemic harm from the use of current spermicides, chiefly nonoxynol-9 or its close relatives. Experience now spans over 70 years. In 1985 a review of 14 studies found no established link with congenital malformations and spontaneous abortions. Occasionally a sensitivity to spermicide arises. Direct local irritation may also occur, particularly if nonoxynol-9 is used very frequently (as by prostitutes). This effect has recently ended the advice to use it as an adjunctive virucide, although in normal use it remains entirely acceptable as a spermicide.

There is a great unmet need for an effective user-friendly female-controlled virucide/spermicide. Research continues.

Methods based on fertility awareness

These are now a more realistic option for many couples, particularly with the advent of Persona (Figure 21). A combination of mini-laboratory and micro-computer, this displays the 'safe' (green) and 'unsafe' (red) days of a woman's cycle based on measurements of her urinary oestrone-3-glucuronide and luteinizing hormone. With (in most couples) only 8–10 'unsafe' days being signalled per cycle, and preliminary data from the manufacturer (not yet fully confirmed) suggesting a failure rate of about

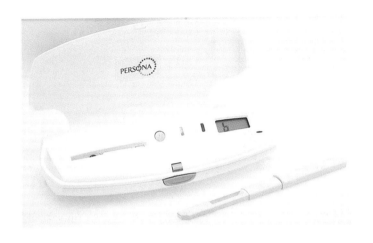

Figure 21
Persona (by courtesy of Unipath Ltd).

6/100 woman-years in the first year of consistent use, this is a welcome new contraceptive option for suitable couples.

'Suitable' must, of course, include acceptance of that estimated 1:17 risk of conceiving in the first year. For greater efficacy, couples can be advised to use condoms on the pre-ovulatory 'green days', to abstain on all 'red days' and to have unprotected intercourse only in the post-ovulatory green phase.

If the method is to be used after pregnancy or *any* hormone treatment — even just one course of hormonal emergency contraception — there must first be two normal cycles of the acceptable length (23–35 days).

See also p. 63 for the lactational amenorrhoea method (LAM), another 'natural' option for some to consider — up to 6 months postpartum.

Appendix

Use of licensed products in an unlicensed way

This is quite often necessary for optimal contraceptive care, and is legitimate provided certain criteria are observed. These are well established (See Mann R. In: Goldberg A, Dodds-Smith I, eds, *Pharmaceutical Medicine and the Law*. London: RCP, 1991:103–110).

The prescribing physician must:

- Adopt a practice endorsed by a responsible body of professional opinion
- Ensure good practice, including follow-up, to comply with professional indemnity requirements. *NB This will often mean the doctor providing dedicated written materials because the manufacturer's insert does not apply*
- **Explain to the individual that it is an unlicensed prescription**
- Give a clear account of the risks and the benefits
- **Obtain informed (verbal) consent and record this and the discussion in full**
- **Keep a separate record of the patient's details**

This is generally termed 'named patient prescribing'.

Some common examples (there are others):

- Advising use of more than one pill per day: when enzyme-inducers are being used with COC (p. 55) or POP (p. 64), or POEC (p. 102); or two POPs daily in the obese young woman (p. 62)
- Use of 'add-back' oestrogen along with Depo Provera (p. 71) to treat diagnosed hypo-oestrogenism
- Use of copper IUDs for longer than licensed, particularly above age 40 (pp. 90–91)
- Insertion of the LNG IUS in a woman who has been sterilized (if the woman herself currently needs or may at any time in the future need contraception it is already licensed, even if her main current problem is menorrhagia, p. 96)
- Use of the LNG IUS as part of hormone replacement therapy (p. 96)
- Use of POEC beyond 72 hours after the earliest exposure *or* more than once in a cycle (pp. 101, 105), but before implantation

Equivalent proprietary names for combined pills worldwide

The following list gives details of some equivalent proprietary names used worldwide which are identical or very similar to UK 'preferred' brands*. Only pills containing less than 50 µg oestrogen are included, and all so-called 'sequential' pills are omitted. (*Note:* occasionally the same or a very similar name is used in different countries for quite different formulations (e.g. Brevinor), so formulations should be carefully checked against that of any previously used packets.) Those brands available in the UK are shown in *italics*.

Phasic pills: for comparison with the monophasics the *average daily* doses given in the UK brands are given in Table 3 (p. 19).

*Based on *Directory of Hormonal Contraceptives* (1996) 3rd edn, compiled by Ronald Kleinman and published by the International Planned Parenthood Federation — see this for a more comprehensive list, including POPs.

Abbreviations

Oestrogens: EE, ethyinyloestradiol. *Progestogens:* NGM, norgestimate; GSD, gestodene; DSG, desogestrel; LNG, levonorgestrel; NET, norethisterone (norethindrone in North America). *Also relatives of NET:* NEA, norethisterone acetate.

Group A (norgestimate, NGM)

EE 35 µg + NGM 250 µg Anele, *Cilest*, Effiprev, Effiprev 35, Ortho-Cyclen

Group B (gestodene, GSD)

EE 35 µg + GSD 75 µg Ciclomex, Evacin, Femodeen, Femoden, *Femodene*, *Femodene ED*, Femovan, Ginera, Ginoden, Gynera, Gynovin, *Minulet*, Minulette, Moneva, Myvlar

EE 20 µg + GSD 75 µg *Femodette*, Harmonet, Meliane

Triphasic formula (EE 30 µg + GSD 50 µg; EE 40 µg + GSD 70 µg; EE 30 µg + GSD 100 µg) Milvane, Phaeva, *Triadene*, Triciclomex, Tri-Femoden, Trigynera, Tri-Gynera, Trigynovin, *Tri-Minulet*, Triodeen, Trioden, Triodena, Triodene

Group C (desogestrel, DSG)

EE 30 µg + DSG 150 µg Cycléane-30, Desogen, Desolett, Frilavon, *Marvelon*, Marviol, Microdiol, Novelon, Ortho-Cept, Planum, Practil, Prevenon, Varnoline

EE 20 µg + DSG 150 µg Cycléane-20, Lovelle, Marvellon 20, *Mercilon*, Microdosis, Myralon, Securgin, Segurin

Group D (levonorgestrel, LNG)

EE 30 µg + LNG 150 µg Ciclo, Ciclon, Combination 3, Contraceptive LD, Duofem*, Egogyn, Egogyn 30, Femigoa,

*These pills also contain dextronorgestrel (non-contraceptive).

Femranette mikro, Follimin, Gynatrol, Levlen, Levo-norgestrel Pill, Levora, Lo-Femenal*, Lo-Gentrol*, Lo-Ovral*, Lo/Ovral*, Lo-Rondal*, Lorsax, Mala D, Microgest, Microginon 30, Microgyn, *Microgynon 30*, *Microgynon 30 ED*, Microvlar, Minibora, Minidril, Minigynon 30, Minivlar, Min-Ovral*, Mithuri, Neo-Gentrol 150/30, Neomonovar, Neovletta, Nordet, Nordette 150/30, Norgestrel Pill*, Norgy-lene, Norvetal, Ologyn-Micro, Ovoplex 30/150, Ovoplexin, Ovral L*, Ovranet, *Ovranette*, Riget, Rigevidon, Sexcon, Stediril-d 150/30, Stediril-30, Stediril-M, Suginor

EE 20 µg + **LNG 100 µg** Alesse, Balancelle, Loette, Leios, *Microgynon 20 (new)*, Micro-Levlen, Miranova

Triphasic formula (EE 30 µg + **LNG 50 µg; EE 40 µg** + **LNG 75 µg; EE 30 µg** + **LNG 125 µg)** Fironetta, Levordiol, *Logynon*, *Logynon ED*, Modutrol, Triagynon, Tri-ciclor, Triette, Trigoa, Trigynon, Trikvilar, Tri-Levlen, *Trinor-diol*, Trionetta, Triovlar, Triphasil, Triquilar, Triquilar ED, Tri-Regol, Trisiston, Tri-Stediril, Triviclor, Trolit

Group E (norethisterone, NET)
EE 35 µg + **NET 1000 µg** Brevicon 1, Brevinor-1, Genora 1/35, Gynex 1/35E, Intercon 1/35, Jenest, Kanchan, Mem-brettes, NEE 1/35, Nelova 1+35E, Neocon, Neo-Norinyl, Norcept-E1/35, Norethin 1/35E, *Norimin*, Norimin-1, Norinyl 1/35, Norquest, Ortho 1+35, Ortho Novum 1/35, Ovysmen 1/35, Secure

EE 35 µg + **NET 500 µg** Brevicon, *Brevinor*, Conceplan mite, Genora 0.5/35, Gynex 0.5/35E, Intercon 5/35, Mikro Plan, Moda Con, Modacon, Modicon, NEE 0.5/35, Nelova 0.5/35E, Neo-Ovopausine, Nilocan, Norminest, Orthonett-Novum, Ovacon, *Ovysmen*, Ovysmen 0.5/35, Perle LD

EE 30 µg + **NEA 1500 µg** *Loestrin 30*, Loestrin 1.5/30, Logest 1.5/30, Minestril-30, Zorane 1.5/30

EE 20 µg + NEA 1000 µg Loestrin, *Loestrin 20*, Loestrin 1/20, Lostrin 1/20, Minestril-20, Minestrin 1/20, Norgest, Zorane 1/20

Triphasic formula (EE 35 µg + NET 500 µg; EE 35 µg + NET 750 µg; EE 35 µg + NET 1000 µg) Ortho 777, Ortho-Novum 777, Triella, *TriNovum*

Triphasic formula (EE 35 µg + NET 500 µg; EE 35 µg + NET 1000 µg; EE 35 µg + NET 500 µg) Improvil, Synfase, *Synphase*, Tri-Norinyl

Further reading

Cooper E, Guillebaud J (1999) *Sexuality and Disability*. Abingdon: Radcliffe Medical.

Guillebaud J (1999) *Contraception — Your Questions Answered*, 3rd edn. Edinburgh: Churchill Livingstone.

Guillebaud J (1997) *The Pill*, 5th edn. Oxford: Oxford University Press.

Kubba A, Sanfilippo J, Hampton N (1999) *Contraception and Office Gynecology*. London: WB Saunders.

Loudon N (2000) *Handbook of Family Planning*,* 4th edn. Edinburgh: Churchill Livingstone.

McPherson A, Waller D (1997) *Women's Problems in General Practice*,* 4th edn. Oxford: Oxford University Press.

Montford H, Skrine R (1993) *Contraceptive Care. Meeting Individual Needs* (Psychosexual Medicine series 6).* London: Chapman & Hall.

* With references.

Many more relevant book titles, videos and useful patient leaflets concerning all methods can be obtained by easy mail order. Contact 'FPA Direct', Unit 9, Ledgers Close, Littlemore, Oxford OX4 5JS, (tel 01865 719418; fax 01865 748746). Leaflets and instructions in languages other than English are also obtainable from the FPA and the International Planned Parenthood Federation, Regent's College, Inner Circle, Regent's Park, London NW1 4NS, and also through some manufacturers.

Index